Annals of the ICRP

ICRP PUBLICATION 140

Radiological Protection in Therapy with Radiopharmaceuticals

Editor-in-Chief
C.H. CLEMENT

Associate Editor
H. FUJITA

Authors on behalf of ICRP
Y. Yonekura, S. Mattsson, G. Flux, W.E. Bolch, L.T. Dauer,
D.R. Fisher, M. Lassmann, S. Palm, M. Hosono,
M. Doruff, C. Divgi, P. Zanzonico

PUBLISHED FOR

The International Commission on Radiological Protection

by

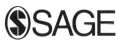

Please cite this issue as 'ICRP, 2019. Radiological protection
in therapy with radiopharmaceuticals. ICRP Publication 140.
Ann. ICRP 48(1).'

CONTENTS

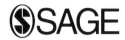
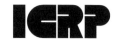

ICRP Publication 140

Guest Editorial

RADIOLOGICAL PROTECTION IN THERAPY WITH RADIOPHARMACEUTICALS

Nuclear medicine is the medical application of radioactive tracer technology invented by Hevesy and Paneth in 1913. Radiopharmaceuticals are chemical and biological substances labelled with a radioisotope and approved as drugs for human medical use by the national authority.

Pharmaceuticals that accumulate selectively in a tissue, organ, or lesion through physiological and metabolic processes are chosen to be labelled with radioisotopes. Due to the very small quantity of pharmaceutical labelled with a very large amount of radioactivity (high specific activity), radiopharmaceuticals do not reveal effects as drugs. Thus, radiopharmaceuticals are used to deliver radioisotopes to specific parts of the body for diagnostic and therapeutic purposes with radiation.

The distribution of a radioisotope and its temporal changes in the body can be traced by external measurement of emitted gamma radiation. The distribution can be displayed as images with quantified radioactivity, which are used for diagnosis, therapy planning, and evaluation of treatment effects. Beta- and alpha-radiation-emitting radioisotopes that accumulate in a lesion such as cancer can destroy cells by focused irradiation of the pathological tissues. This mechanism is used for therapy. The efficient use of radiopharmaceuticals for both diagnosis and therapy using alpha, beta, and gamma radionuclides is called 'theranostics'.

In the 1940s, the first reports of the use of radioactive iodine to treat diseases of the thyroid, and radioactive phosphorus to treat leukaemia were greeted with great enthusiasm by the medical profession and the public. These classic findings were immediately recognised as forerunners of a whole series of similar uses of radioactive 'magic bullets' (Wagner, 2006). Even today, radioiodine therapy of hyperthyroidism and thyroid cancers is increasingly used in Japan and elsewhere. Bone-seeking agents labelled with ^{89}Sr or ^{153}Sm have been used for relief of intractable bone pain. Alpha-emitting ^{223}Ra-dichloride has been shown to reduce pain and extend survival of patients with multiple bone metastases. The treatment of metastatic endocrine tumours using radiopharmaceuticals that bind to hormone receptors such as somatostatin receptors has been widely used in Europe, and is expected to be approved in Japan.

Radioimmunotherapy targeting cancer-related antigens, such as prostate-specific membrane antigen, has been investigated for clinical uses using antibodies labelled with beta emitters such as ^{131}I, ^{90}Y, ^{153}Sm, and ^{177}Lu, as well as alpha emitters such as ^{211}At, ^{213}Bi, and ^{225}Ac. Theranostics is a new medical science that combines the diagnostic properties of antibodies labelled with photon-emitting radionuclides with therapeutic alpha- and beta-emitting radionuclides.

Medical use of technologies for radiopharmaceutical targeting of pathologic tissues in cancer treatment has been expanding worldwide. The number of patients who receive radiopharmaceutical therapy has doubled in the past 10 years in Japan.

Radiological protection in radiopharmaceutical therapy has unique aspects because unsealed radionuclides are used with much greater activities than commonly employed in diagnostic nuclear medicine. These greater activities may require hospitalisation of patients in wards specifically designed and equipped with special shielding and contamination control. The criteria for the release of patients or treatment as outpatients must be determined based on potential dose to family and friends.

Patients who receive radiopharmaceuticals for therapeutic purposes become radiation sources with larger doses and for longer periods compared with those who receive radiopharmaceuticals for diagnostic purposes. Special protective measures must be taken with regards to contact with other people, especially children and pregnant women. If these patients travel or pass by radiation monitors, alerts may be activated. Therefore, patients should carry relevant documents issued by the hospitals. Breast feeding must be stopped and conception should be avoided for certain periods of time. Special considerations for radiological protection are also necessary if radioactive patients are on dialysis.

Hospital staff who deal with radiopharmaceutical therapy need special training and experience in safety measures, in addition to those for regular radiation workers, to avoid contamination from unsealed radiation sources. They also need to know how to decontaminate in case of contamination. Special care is required to contain contamination within controlled areas.

For decades, ICRP has developed dose coefficients and other guidance related to calculating doses to patients undergoing procedures using radiopharmaceuticals. Most recently, these have been summarised in *Publication 128* (ICRP, 2015a).

In the current publication, ICRP provides recommendations on radiological protection of patients, staff, and members of the public relating to radiopharmaceutical therapy. Nuclear medicine physicians who practice radiopharmaceutical therapy, doctors who prescribe it, and other hospital staff who are involved need to be familiar with radiological protection considerations for patients and workers.

In case of nuclear or radiological accidents or malicious acts, people with internal exposure to radioactive materials must be hospitalised for radiation dose estimation and treatment. The most appropriate facilities for these purposes are rooms designed specifically for radiopharmaceutical therapy. Medical personnel trained in the care of therapy patients may also be excellent specialists for dealing with other types of radiological emergencies. Staff should receive training with regular exercises to ensure that they are prepared for unanticipated nuclear or radiological medical emergencies.

YASUHITO SASAKI
ICRP MAIN COMMISSION MEMBER (2001-2009)

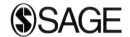
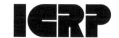

RADIOLOGICAL PROTECTION IN THERAPY WITH RADIOPHARMACEUTICALS

ICRP PUBLICATION 140

Approved by the Commission in November 2018

Abstract–Radiopharmaceuticals are increasingly used for the treatment of various cancers with novel radionuclides, compounds, tracer molecules, and administration techniques. The goal of radiation therapy, including therapy with radiopharmaceuticals, is to optimise the relationship between tumour control probability and potential complications in normal organs and tissues. Essential to this optimisation is the ability to quantify the radiation doses delivered to both tumours and normal tissues. This publication provides an overview of therapeutic procedures and a framework for calculating radiation doses for various treatment approaches. In radiopharmaceutical therapy, the absorbed dose to an organ or tissue is governed by radiopharmaceutical uptake, retention in and clearance from the various organs and tissues of the body, together with radionuclide physical half-life. Biokinetic parameters are determined by direct measurements made using techniques that vary in complexity. For treatment planning, absorbed dose calculations are usually performed prior to therapy using a trace-labelled diagnostic administration, or retrospective dosimetry may be performed on the basis of the activity already administered following each therapeutic administration. Uncertainty analyses provide additional information about sources of bias and random variation and their magnitudes; these analyses show the reliability and quality of absorbed dose calculations. Effective dose can provide an approximate measure of lifetime risk of detriment attributable to the stochastic effects of radiation exposure, principally cancer, but effective dose does not predict future cancer incidence for an individual and does not apply to short-term deterministic effects associated with radiopharmaceutical therapy. Accident prevention in radiation therapy should be an integral part of the design of facilities, equipment, and administration procedures. Minimisation of staff exposures includes consideration of equipment design, proper shielding and handling of sources, and personal protective equipment and tools, as well as education and training to promote awareness and engagement in radiological protection. The decision to hold or release a patient after radiopharmaceutical therapy should account for potential radiation dose to members of the public and carers that may result from residual radioactivity in the patient. In these situations, specific radiological protection guidance should be provided to patients and carers.

© 2019 ICRP. Published by SAGE.

Keywords: Radiopharmaceutical therapy; Radionuclide; Dose estimation; Radiological protection

MAIN POINTS

- Treatment with radiopharmaceuticals requires administration protocols that justify and optimise the treatment. Individual absorbed dose estimates should be performed for treatment planning and for postadministration verification of doses to tumours and normal tissues.

- Special consideration should be given to pregnant women and children exposed to ionising radiation. Pregnancy is usually contraindicated in radiopharmaceutical therapy. Breast feeding should be discontinued in patients receiving radiopharmaceutical therapy.

- Radiation sources used in radiopharmaceutical therapy can contribute to exposures to medical personnel and others who may spend time within or adjacent to rooms that contain such sources. Meaningful radiation dose reduction and contamination control can be achieved through the use of appropriate procedures, and facility and room design, including shielding where appropriate, as well as education and training to promote awareness and engagement in radiological protection. Accident prevention and review of safe practices in radiopharmaceutical therapy should be an integral part of the design of facilities, equipment, and administration procedures.

- Medical practitioners should provide all necessary medical care consistent with the radiological protection principles of justification and optimisation. Radiological protection actions should not prevent or delay life-saving medical procedures or surgery in the event that they may be required for medical care. Staff should be informed and trained with respect to patient radiation levels.

- The decision to hospitalise or release a patient after therapy should be made based on existing guidance and regulations, as well as on the individual patient's situation, considering factors such as the residual activity in the patient, the patient's wishes, and family considerations (particularly the presence of children or pregnant family members). Information to guide radiological protection at home should be provided to patients and carers.

1. INTRODUCTION

(1) In radiation therapy, cancer is treated to preserve life and to improve the quality of life of the patient. While radiation therapy focuses on treating the malignancy, absorbed doses delivered to normal organs and tissues should be minimised to limit adverse tissue reactions. Current ICRP recommendations related to therapy with radiopharmaceuticals are found in *Publications 73* (ICRP, 1996a), *94* (ICRP, 2004), *103* (ICRP, 2007a), and *105* (ICRP, 2007b).

(2) The medical community currently does not have adequate resources for the collection of useful biokinetic or dosimetric data for such procedures. However, quantitative imaging and dosimetry should be the basis for treatment planning for radiopharmaceutical therapy,[1] just as they are for external-beam radiotherapy.

(3) Collection and review of the existing information and literature will help to optimise therapeutic use of radiopharmaceuticals, particularly for newer approaches. It is essential to alert the community to the variation in patient biokinetics at therapeutic levels of activity. This information can facilitate the introduction of new radiopharmaceuticals, particularly with regard to the levels of administered activity prescribed.

(4) Many publications deal with absorbed doses delivered to critical organs and tumours. These include details on the biokinetics of uptake and retention. It would be valuable if a greater amount of biokinetic information could be provided from the increasing number of studies that are being performed. It would also be beneficial to assess the integrity of data gathered from descriptions of the methods used to acquire the data.

(5) This publication details a framework to perform individualised dosimetry to plan therapeutic procedures and to verify the absorbed dose delivered.

(6) Therapeutic radiopharmaceuticals typically exhibit large differences in biokinetics from one patient to another. Personalised dosimetry is essential to ascertain individual radiopharmaceutical biokinetics to ensure that a subsequent therapy administration does not exceed organ or tissue tolerance levels. The practice and optimisation of radiopharmaceutical therapy practice and optimisation requires different competencies, including medical physicists, nuclear medicine technologists, nuclear medicine physicians, endocrinologists, and oncologists.

(7) The target audience of this publication includes nuclear medicine physicians and oncologists, medical physicists, clinicians, practitioners and prescribers, referrers, radiopharmacists, nuclear medicine technologists, radiographers, radiation protection officers, regulatory authorities, medical and scientific societies, industry, patients, patient advocacy groups, and public protection officials.

---

[1]Therapy with radiopharmaceuticals is referred to by many synonymous terms, including 'targeted radionuclide therapy', 'unsealed source therapy', 'systemic radiation therapy', and 'molecular radiotherapy'. In this publication, the generic term 'radiopharmaceutical therapy' is used for consistency with other ICRP and ICRU publications.

2. RADIOPHARMACEUTICAL THERAPY METHODS: JUSTIFICATION AND OPTIMISATION

2.1. Introduction

(8) Radiopharmaceutical therapy is a complex procedure, encompassing a wide range of radionuclides, different targeting mechanisms, and various methods of administration. Each radiotherapeutic procedure presents a unique set of challenges for dosimetric calculations, related to quantitative imaging, absorbed dose calculations, and considerations of normal tissue detriment. The need for a highly multidisciplinary approach and the relatively small number of patients treated has resulted in a lack of development within the field compared with that for external-beam radiotherapy (NCRP, 2006).

(9) The objectives of treatment with radiopharmaceuticals are often palliative, as in the case of beta emitters for bone metastases. Complete responses are common only in limited cases, such as for the ablation of thyroid remnants following thyroidectomy. In the majority of treatments, a range of responses are seen.

(10) Radionuclide therapy using ^{131}I-iodide for the treatment of thyrotoxicosis and thyroid cancer, and ^{32}P-phosphate for polycythaemia and palliation of bone pain has been practised for more than 70 years. Radionuclide therapy is increasingly used for treating various tumours using several novel radionuclides, compounds, tracer molecules, and application techniques. Examples of recently developed methods used in clinical practice are ^{177}Lu-labelled peptides for treating neuroendocrine tumours and ^{223}Ra-dichloride for treating bone metastases from prostate cancer.

(11) Clinical introduction of a new radiotherapeutic method involves the development of administration protocols that justify and optimise the treatment.

(12) Many new radiopharmaceuticals are being developed. Each new agent must be considered separately, and the potential benefits and risks involved must be considered in relation to safety and efficacy, individual patient status, and the aim of treatment.

(13) Records of the specifics of therapy with unsealed radionuclides should be maintained. Data concerned with absorbed dose planning and activities of administered radiopharmaceuticals should always be included in the patient's medical records.

(14) Dose coefficients presented in *Publications 106* (ICRP, 2008), *128* (ICRP, 2015a), *53* (ICRP, 1987), and *80* (ICRP, 1998) are intended for diagnostic nuclear medicine and not for therapeutic applications. The use of radiopharmaceuticals for therapy requires more detailed, patient-specific dosimetry for treatment planning, with dosimetry for both tumours and normal organs and tissues.

2.2. Treatment of hyperthyroidism and other benign thyroid conditions

(15) ^{131}I-iodide, first used in the 1940s (Seidlin et al., 1946), is a routine treatment for diffuse or nodular toxic goitre, hyperthyroidism, or large non-toxic goitre (Leiter et al.,

1946). The treatment is usually performed by oral administration of a capsule containing ^{131}I-iodide, but ^{131}I solution is also used for individualised administration of the activity. Radioactive iodine accumulates in the thyroid gland, and beta particles emitted by ^{131}I destroy the cells of the thyroid gland. Although this is established as a first-line treatment, there is little consensus concerning treatment regimens, and there is ongoing controversy over the aims of treatment.

2.2.1. Aim of treatment

(16) The aim of treatment is to destroy the cells of the thyroid gland and to suppress the hyperactive thyroid function to render the patient euthyroid or hypothyroid.

2.2.2. Treatment protocols

(17) Treatment protocols fall into three categories according to the treatment objective.

- An administration of a fixed activity with the aim to render patients hypothyroid within a short period of time, whereupon patients continue on life-long thyroid replacement hormones (RCP, 2007).
- A personalised approach to inducing hypothyroidism to achieve a prompt response albeit with the minimal administered activity necessary (Kobe et al., 2008; Stokkel et al., 2010; Schiavo et al., 2011).
- A personalised approach with the aim of rendering patients euthyroid where possible, and to delay the need for supplementary medication (Flower et al., 1994; Howarth et al., 2001).

2.2.3. Radiation dose to friends and family

(18) Radioiodine is primarily excreted via urine, but also through faeces and perspiration (Hänscheid et al., 2013; ICRP, 2015a,b). The mean effective half-time for excretion of ^{131}I from the thyroid is approximately 5 days, although this has been shown to vary widely. Radiation dose assessments should be performed for individual treatments, taking into account patient-specific factors. Detailed written guidance for reducing exposure from the patient should be provided to the patient and their family.

2.2.4. Radiation dose to staff

(19) The levels of activity administered for treatment of benign thyroid conditions are substantially less than those administered for ablation or therapeutic procedures, and greater than those administered for diagnostic studies. Occupational doses should be determined for staff members who work with ^{131}I, and it may be important to track thyroid doses for radiopharmacists who handle ^{131}I.

2.2.5. Patient organ dosimetry

(20) The role of internal dosimetry in the management of benign thyroid disease with radioiodine remains a matter of debate. In some cases, activities are administered without dosimetric consideration, while in other cases, dosimetry is performed to guide treatment (Stokkel et al., 2010). Advances in quantitative imaging and dosimetry enable more precise dosimetric calculations that may take into account volume and sequential retention measurements acquired from ^{131}I or ^{123}I single-photon emission computed tomography (SPECT), and [124]I positron emission tomography (PET) (Merrill et al., 2011). Dosimetric guidelines have been published by the European Association of Nuclear Medicine (EANM) (Hänscheid et al., 2013).

2.2.6. Risks to patients

(21) As with all therapeutic procedures, pregnancy and breast feeding are contra-indicated for treatment, and patients should avoid conception for 4–6 months (see Sections 5.3.3 and 5.3.4). Identification of any patient who may be pregnant is crucial as ^{131}I-iodide is taken up by the fetal thyroid from 8–10 weeks post conception, and doses to the fetal thyroid can result in permanent hypothyroidism and a risk for severe physical and mental retardation due to deficiency of thyroid hormones (Berg et al., 1998). Patients to be treated with radioactive iodine should not undergo tests with iodinated contrast media within 2 months prior to the therapy, due to the risk of iodine blockage and low uptake of radioactive iodine (Luster et al., 2008).

2.2.7. Recommendations

(22) At present, there are no standardised protocols for thyroid disease treatment, which reflects the lack of evidence base for best practice. A fixed activity administration, without dosimetric calculations, while convenient for many centres, results in the administration of higher activities than is necessary for effective treatment of benign thyroid disease (Jönsson and Mattsson, 2004; Sisson et al., 2007).

(23) In principle, a personalised approach based on patient-specific measurements can ensure the administration of minimal effective activity, thereby minimising the potential for long-term risks and the radiation doses delivered to staff, family, and comforters and carers. A personalised dosimetric approach may provide the potential to render patients euthyroid where this may be desired. There have been a limited number of trials to date to investigate the potential of a personalised approach to treatment (Leslie et al., 2003), and further trials are needed to determine the relationship between the absorbed doses delivered to the thyroid and normal organs and outcome. Such trials should be stratified according to the volume of the thyroid, initial uptake, and retention (Howarth et al., 2001; Reinhardt et al., 2002).

2.3. Treatment of differentiated thyroid cancer

(24) ^{131}I-iodide has become a treatment of choice for the ablation and therapy of papillary and follicular thyroid cancer. Patients are typically given a low iodine diet prior to administration (Haugen et al., 2016). Some guidelines now also indicate the use of recombinant human thyroid-stimulating hormone (Thyrogen, Genzyme Corp., Cambridge, MA, USA) as an adjunctive treatment to stimulate uptake for radioiodine ablation of thyroid tissue remnants in patients who have undergone near-total or total thyroidectomy for well-differentiated thyroid cancer and who have evidence of distant metastatic thyroid cancer. Subsequent administrations are given for further therapy of recurrent or persistent disease, particularly in the case of metastatic spread. Administrations are continued, typically at 6–8-month intervals, until patients become iodine negative or fail to show a therapeutic response.

(25) Management guidelines have been published for adult patients with thyroid nodules and differentiated thyroid cancer (Silberstein et al., 2012; Haugen et al., 2016), and for the diagnosis and management of thyroid disease during pregnancy and the postpartum period (Alexander et al., 2017).

2.3.1. Aim of treatment

(26) For ablation, the aim of treatment is to eradicate residual normal thyroid tissue and malignant tissue. Several professional medical societies have provided management guidelines for patients with thyroid nodules and differentiated thyroid cancer (Luster et al., 2008; Haugen et al., 2016). For some staging criteria, opinions differ regarding the therapeutic effectiveness of radioiodine (Perros et al., 2014). In some cases, persistent yet stable disease is expected.

2.3.2. Treatment protocols

(27) In spite of the widespread use of this treatment over many decades, the level of evidence for optimal radioiodine treatments is low (Luster et al., 2008). No multi-centre trials have been conducted to date to establish the optimal activity to administer for ablation or subsequent therapeutic procedures. Consequently, guidelines do not give strong recommendations regarding optimised levels of administration.

(28) In recent years, the UK HiLo trial and the French ESTIMABL trial demonstrated that 1.1 GBq ^{131}I is as effective as 3.7 GBq for ablation in low- or intermediate-risk patients, although the interpretation of these results is debated. An ongoing discussion concerns whether radioiodine should be administered at all in low-risk patients (Mallick et al., 2012b; Schlumberger et al., 2012; Haugen et al., 2016).

(29) In the absence of trial-based evidence, activity schedules have been proposed to maximise therapy effectiveness and to minimise the likelihood of secondary malignancies.

(30) To date, there have been no randomised controlled clinical trials for the treatment of children with differentiated thyroid cancer, and only one set of guidelines has been written (Francis et al., 2015). Administrations for radioiodine ablation in children vary widely. Activity may be adjusted by body weight (usually 1.85–7.4 MBq kg^{-1}), by body surface area, or by age (Jarzab et al., 2005; Luster et al., 2008). A hybrid approach of combining 24-h-uptake measurements with body weight is favoured by the German procedure guidelines (Franzius et al., 2007).

(31) Treatment protocols for therapy administrations also vary. Fixed activities of 1.1–11.0 GBq have been administered to children, as well as a range of activities based on body weight (Jarzab et al., 2005; Franzius et al., 2007; Luster et al., 2008; Verburg et al., 2011).

2.3.3. Radiation dose to friends and family

(32) Retention and excretion of radioiodine vary among patients. The mean effective half-time for ^{131}I excretion after total thyroidectomy is less than that for hyperthyroidism (Hänscheid et al., 2006; Remy et al., 2008). Written guidance should be provided to the patient, taking into account their family circumstances, and comforter and carer consent is required if in close contact with the patient.

(33) Patients undergoing treatment may require hospitalisation following administration, according to national patient release regulations. The decision to hospitalise or to release a patient should be determined on an individual basis according to calculations of potential radiation doses to family and members of the public.

2.3.4. Radiation dose to staff

(34) As with all procedures involving radiotherapeutics, standard precautions should be taken with the principle of dose limitation. As patients are hospitalised, there are risks to different groups of staff, including nurses, technologists, physicists, and physicians, and staff doses should be monitored.

2.3.5. Patient organ dosimetry

(35) Fixed administration protocols result in the delivery of a very wide range of absorbed doses to target thyroid tissues (Flux et al., 2010).

(36) Seidlin et al. (1946) calculated the cumulative absorbed doses to metastases. Further studies have used a blood absorbed dose of 2 Gy as a surrogate biomarker for marrow toxicity (Benua et al., 1962), 300 Gy to ablate thyroid remnant tissue, and 80 Gy to eradicate lymph node metastases (Maxon et al., 1992).

(37) Dosimetric studies show significant correlations between the absorbed doses delivered and therapeutic response (Strigari et al., 2014), and dosimetric guidelines have been published by EANM (Lassmann et al., 2008).

2.3.6. Risks to patients

(38) As with all therapeutic procedures, pregnancy and breast feeding are contra-indicated. Conception advice is given according to national guidelines (see Section 5.3.6). A range of side effects can arise from administration of radioiodine, the most common being sialadenitis and gastritis (Luster et al., 2008). A single administration of radioiodine can induce permanent xerostomia and can increase the risk of salivary malignancies (Klubo-Gwiezdzinska et al., 2010; Lee, 2010). A decline in leukocytes and platelets may also be seen. Pulmonary fibrosis has been observed in patients with thyroid-origin lung metastases (Haugen et al., 2016). Patients to be treated with radioactive iodine should not undergo tests with iodinated contrast media within 2 months prior to therapy due to the risk of iodine blockage with low uptake of radioactive iodine (Luster et al., 2008).

(39) Children and young people treated with radioiodine for differentiated thyroid cancer are likely to have a significantly longer survival than is the case for adults, although 2% have long-term cause-specific mortality. Children with pulmonary metastases may develop stable disease following administration of radioiodine (Vassilopoulou-Sellin et al., 1993; Pawelczak et al., 2010). Long-term follow-up of children treated with radioiodine for differentiated thyroid cancer has shown an increase in secondary malignancies (Rubino et al., 2003; Brown et al., 2008; Hay et al., 2010; Francis et al., 2015). The risk of leukaemia increases with increasing cumulative activity, and patients are more likely to develop secondary malignancies in the bladder, colorectal system, breast, and salivary glands.

2.3.7. Recommendations

(40) The 10-year overall cause-specific survival for differentiated thyroid cancer is approximately 85% (Luster et al., 2008), depending on age, volume of disease, and metastatic spread (Mallick et al., 2012a). On the other hand, the 10-year survival in cases with distant metastases is only 25–40%, indicating the need for stratification in treatment planning. The recurrence rate can be as high as 10–30%. Insufficient treatment may necessitate further therapy at the risk of continuing progression and the development of iodine negativity. Excess radiation delivered to normal tissues is associated with potential side effects and some risk of secondary malignancies.

(41) The obvious benefit of complete cure and the need to minimise the potential for secondary malignancies show the importance of dosimetry for each treatment. This is particularly relevant for children and young people, and for high-risk patients. Further studies are needed to investigate the role of pretherapy dosimetry planning, taking into account the possibility of stunning, whereby uptake of activity for therapy may be reduced. Thyroid stunning is a clinical observation in which exposure of a patient to diagnostic amounts of ^{131}I has been described to alter the

ability of differentiated thyroid carcinoma or remnants of thyroid tissue after thyroidectomy to assimilate administered [131]I.

2.4. Treatment of polycythaemia vera and essential thrombocythaemia

(42) ^{32}P-phosphate was first used to treat polycythaemia vera and essential thrombocythaemia approximately 70 years ago. Polycythaemia vera and essential thrombocythaemia are chronic progressive myeloproliferative disorders characterised by overproduction of erythrocytes and thrombocytes, respectively. Other disease features include leukocytosis, splenomegaly, thrombohaemorrhagic complications, vasomotor disturbances, pruritus, and a risk of disease progression into acute myeloid leukaemia or myelofibrosis. With the introduction of agents such as hydroxycarbamide, interferon, and anagrelide, the role of ^{32}P has diminished. Today, polycythaemia vera and essential thrombocythaemia remain the only myeloproliferative conditions treated by ^{32}P-phosphate.

2.4.1. Aim of treatment

(43) ^{32}P is actively incorporated into DNA of rapidly proliferating cells. Treatment suppresses blood cell production by irradiating bone marrow. Beta radiation from ^{32}P suppresses hyperproliferative cell lines. Despite alternative treatments, elderly patients with polycythaemia vera and essential thrombocythaemia respond to oral or intravenous administration of ^{32}P-phosphate (Tennvall and Brans, 2007).

2.4.2. Treatment protocols

(44) ^{32}P-phosphate is administered intravenously or orally. The administered activity is 74–111 MBq m^{-2} body surface with a maximum upper activity limit of 185 MBq, or a slightly higher activity of 3.7 MBq kg^{-1} body weight with a maximum upper activity limit of 260 MBq. A decrease in activity of 25% in patients aged >80 years is recommended by some investigators. An alternative, dose-escalating approach is to administer a fixed lower activity of 111 MBq. In the absence of an 'adequate response', a second treatment may be given after 3 months with a 25% increase in activity. This procedure of increased activity may be repeated every 3 months until an adequate therapeutic response is obtained. The upper activity limit for a single administration is 260 MBq (Tennvall and Brans, 2007).

2.4.3. Radiation dose to friends and family

(45) For outpatient therapy, the patient and family should be instructed to: (1) avoid prolonged, close contact with young children and pregnant women; (2) sleep in

a separate bed from a partner or children for a few days after return home; and (3) practice good personal hygiene to avoid any external contamination as ^{32}P is excreted in urine for 2–3 weeks after treatment.

2.4.4. Radiation dose to staff

(46) As ^{32}P is a high-energy beta emitter, it is essential to employ plastic and metal shielding during dispensing and injection.

2.4.5. Patient organ dosimetry

(47) Organs with the highest radiation dose are bone endosteum and haemato-poietically active bone marrow, which receive approximately 11 mGy per MBq administered (ICRP, 1987). A typical administration of 100 MBq may impart more than 1 Gy to bone endosteum and active bone marrow.

2.4.6. Risks to patients

(48) Contraindications are pregnancy and breast feeding, and patients should avoid conception. The radiopharmaceutical is not recommended for women of child-bearing age. The incidence of acute myeloid leukaemia 10 years after ^{32}P treatment is approximately 10% (Brandt and Anderson, 1995). Treatment using ^{32}P is therefore usually reserved for patients over the age of 65–70 years.

2.4.7. Recommendations

(49) ^{32}P-phosphate can be used in elderly patients and those for whom alternative treatments such as hydroxyurea, busulphan, interferon-alpha, or anagrelide are not suitable.

2.5. Treatment of skeletal metastases

(50) Treatment of painful skeletal metastases is important for management of cancer patients who are in advanced stages and need palliative care. Painful bone metastases may impair quality of life through limitation of daily activity, restricted mobility, insomnia, and anxiety. Management of bone pain is multi-disciplinary, and may include analgesia, radiation, hormones, chemotherapy, bisphosphonates, and surgery. Localised metastases can be treated with external-beam radiation or surgery. Diffuse bone metastases are usually treated by radiopharmaceuticals, hormones, chemotherapy, and bisphosphonates (Pandit-Taskar et al., 2004).

(51) Beta-emitting radiopharmaceuticals such as ^{89}Sr-chloride and ^{153}Sm-EDTMP (ethylenediamine tetramethylene phosphonate) have been administered for pain relief

in patients with painful skeletal metastases as palliative therapy. [223]Ra-dichloride, an alpha-emitting bone-seeking radiopharmaceutical, has emerged as a radiopharmaceutical therapy agent for castration-resistant prostate cancer with symptomatic bone metastases, and has been shown to prolong overall survival (3–6 months) (Parker et al., 2013; Pandit-Takar et al., 2014).

2.5.1. Aim of treatment

(52) The aim of treatment with beta-emitting radiopharmaceuticals is to control bone pain due to metastases and to improve quality of life in patients suffering from skeletal metastases. These agents are rarely curative. ^{89}Sr-chloride and [153]Sm-EDTMP are approved in some countries for relief of painful skeletal metastases from solid cancers, while [186]Re-HEDP (hydroxyethyledinediphosphonate), [188]Re-HEDP, [117m]Sn-DTPA (diethylenetriamine pentaacetic acid), and ^{177}Lu-EDTMP are under investigation (Finlay et al., 2005; Liepe et al., 2005b; Liepe and Kotzerke, 2007; Shinto et al., 2014; Yousefnia et al., 2015). The mechanism of pain relief by these radiopharmaceuticals is believed to be due to reduction of pressure on neurons. The aim of treatment of [223]Ra-dichloride therapy in prostate cancer patients with bone metastases is to improve quality of life by mitigating pain without use of addictive pain killers while prolonging overall survival.

2.5.2. Treatment protocols

(53) ^{89}Sr-chloride and [153]Sm-EDTMP are approved in several countries and thus have well-established treatment protocols. The recommended dosage of ^{89}Sr-chloride is 148 MBq. Alternatively, a dosage of 1.5–2.2 MBq kg^{-1} body weight may be administered as a single intravenous injection, compared with [153]Sm-EDTMP at an activity per body weight of 37 MBq kg^{-1}. For both radiopharmaceuticals, patients must visit their doctors regularly to ensure that the treatments are having a beneficial effect and to check for unwanted effects including leukocytopenia and thrombocytopenia. Treatment protocols are under study for [186]Re-HEDP, [188]Re-HEDP, [117m]Sn-DTPA, and ^{177}Lu-EDTMP (Pandit-Taskar et al., 2004; Liepe and Kotzerke, 2007; Bodei et al., 2008; D'Angelo et al., 2012; Jie et al., 2013; Thapa et al., 2015).

(54) The approved administered activity per body weight for [223]Ra-dichloride is 55 kBq kg^{-1} given intravenously as one administration every 4 weeks over a period of 6 months.

2.5.3. Radiation dose to friends and family

(55) As activity is excreted mainly through urine for ^{89}Sr-chloride and [153]Sm-EDTMP, and through faeces for [223]Ra-dichloride, care must be taken to ensure that all excreta are disposed of in the sanitary sewer system when a patient is at home. Nappies and other potentially contaminated material should be collected in

specified bags for waste disposal. The specified rubbish bags must be leak proof, and bags containing waste could be returned to the treating facility, as determined by the respective treatment personnel (Sisson et al., 2011). Patients may be hospitalised for a longer period if mentally incompetent and/or incontinent and therefore incapable of following radiation safety instructions and precautions (ICRP, 2004).

2.5.4. Radiation dose to staff

(56) For ^{89}Sr, ^{153}Sm-EDTMP, and ^{223}Ra, patients can receive treatment on an outpatient basis, which is advantageous for ensuring that exposures of staff remain low. Higher irradiation of ^{186}Re-HEDP and ^{188}Re-HEDP results from the gamma emissions. Staff doses should be monitored carefully in all cases. ^{223}Ra-dichloride has been evaluated as safe and straightforward to handle and administer using conventional nuclear medicine equipment (Dauer et al., 2014).

2.5.5. Patient organ dosimetry

(57) ^{89}Sr delivers absorbed doses of 0.2–2 and 0.05–0.3 Gy MBq^{-1} to the bone surfaces adjacent to metastatic sites and to red marrow, respectively (Breen et al., 1992), while ^{153}Sm-EDTMP imparts absorbed doses of 5.3–8.8 and 1.2–2.0 mGy MBq^{-1} to the bone surfaces and red marrow, respectively (Eary et al., 1993). Absorbed dose values may vary depending on individual patient biokinetics and metabolism. The range of absorbed doses of ^{223}Ra-dichloride calculated from Phase 1 study data were 2–13 Gy MBq^{-1} for bone surfaces, while absorbed doses to red marrow were 177–994 and 1–5 mGy MBq^{-1} from bone surfaces and blood activity, respectively (Chittenden et al., 2015).

2.5.6. Risk to patients

(58) Radiopharmaceuticals used for therapy of bone metastases may cause bone marrow suppression, especially in patients with reduced bone marrow reserve who have previously been treated with repeated chemotherapy. A transient rise in bone pain a few days after administration may occur in some patients. Patients with renal dysfunction must undergo careful evaluation prior to treatment because adverse effects including bone marrow suppression may be more serious. Contraindications are pregnancy and breast feeding.

(59) ^{223}Ra has the advantage of sparing much of the marrow from irradiation by virtue of its short-range alpha emissions. Non-haematological toxicities are generally more common than haematologic toxicity and are mild to moderate in intensity; they include diarrhoea, fatigue, nausea, vomiting, and bone pain, some of which are dose-related (Pandit-Taskar et al., 2014). The long-term adverse effects of ^{223}Ra in patients with extended survival are not yet known.

2.5.7. Recommendations

(60) Bone-seeking radiopharmaceuticals have important roles in the management of painful bone metastases by alleviating pain and improving quality of life. Pain relief may last for several months after a single injection. The widely different administration protocols for each agent, that may be fixed or weight-based and may be administered once or multiple times, indicate that optimal treatment protocols are not yet established and that further studies are necessary to this end. In terms of adverse effects, haematological toxicity due to marrow exposure should be taken into account. An investigation of the optimal absorbed dose to deliver for ^{223}Ra would help to determine optimal treatment regimens and identify patients in whom treatment is likely to have little or no benefit. The radiopharmaceuticals are usually administered on an outpatient basis, and standard radiological protection precautions are required.

2.6. Treatment of neuroblastoma in children and young adults

(61) Metaiodobenzylguanidine (mIBG), introduced in the 1980s, is a guanethidine and noradrenaline analogue taken up by cells of the sympathetic nervous system by an active transport process involving the noradrenaline transporter molecule.

(62) Neuroblastoma arises from the neural crest cells involved in development of the nervous system and other tissues. It commonly occurs in the adrenal glands or in the nerve tissue, and can spread to bones and liver. Neuroblastoma accounts for approximately 6% of childhood cancers, with only 67% surviving for ≥ 5 years. ^{131}I-mIBG is most commonly administered in chemorefractory or relapsed patients. Outcomes vary from 30% to 58% (Hoefnagel et al., 1991; Garaventa et al., 1999; Matthay et al., 2007).

2.6.1. Aim of treatment

(63) The aim of treatment is predominantly palliative. A range of responses are seen, including complete responses and downstaging, which may permit further surgery or external-beam radiotherapy (George et al., 2016).

2.6.2. Treatment protocols

(64) Treatment regimens for ^{131}I-mIBG vary widely. There are currently no established guidelines to govern the levels of activity administered. Typically, empirical fixed activities have been administered, comprising multiples of 3.7 GBq (Hoefnagel et al., 1991; Tristam et al., 1996), although weight-based activities have also frequently been administered. Short-term toxicity may correlate with the whole-body absorbed dose, which can therefore act as a surrogate for the absorbed dose delivered to the red marrow. This has led to an alternative approach to fixed activity

administrations, whereby the activities are tailored to deliver a prescribed whole-body absorbed dose (Gaze et al., 2005; Buckley et al., 2009). This can entail two administrations of 555–666 MBq kg^{-1} to deliver a total whole-body absorbed dose of 4 Gy, with peripheral blood stem cell support (Giammarile et al., 2008). There is, similarly, no protocol to govern the number of treatments delivered, and although single treatments have been administered, administrations are sometimes repeated and as many as five administrations have been reported (George et al., 2016).

2.6.3. Radiation dose to friends and family

(65) Precautions must be considered for each patient, taking home circumstances into account. This is particularly relevant for children and young people who may have siblings at home. Excretion is predominantly via the urine, and care must be taken to ensure that all excreta are disposed of in the sanitary sewer system. Written instructions must be provided to patients and their families and carers on discharge from hospital.

2.6.4. Radiation dose to staff

(66) Careful protection procedures are required to minimise radiation from the source and the administered patient. Shielded syringes should be employed during intravenous administration to ensure that extremity doses to medical staff and radio-pharmacists are maintained as low as possible. The use of an automatic injection system will significantly reduce the radiation exposure of staff members (Rushforth et al., 2017). Administration protocols must be carefully considered. Personalised protocols (Gaze et al., 2005; Buckley et al., 2009) can entail extremely high levels of radiation in comparison with other treatments. Nursing staff, in particular, require specific training in radiological protection. Valuable advice related to administration of high-dose ^{131}I-MIBG therapy to children is given by Chu et al. (2016).

2.6.5. Patient organ dosimetry

(67) In contrast to many therapeutic procedures with radiopharmaceuticals, a large number of dosimetric studies have been performed relative to the number of centres that offer ^{131}I-mIBG therapy (Tristam et al., 1996; Matthay et al., 2001; Sudbrock et al., 2010; Flux et al., 2011). The absorbed doses delivered to the whole body, critical organs, and tumours have been reported to vary by an order of magnitude (Matthay et al., 2001; Flux et al., 2011), indicating the important role of personalised dosimetry.

2.6.6. Risks to patients

(68) Acute toxicity is primarily haematological, causing neutropenia, thrombo-cytopenia, and leukocytopenia (Buckley et al., 2009). Thyroid blockade is essential, but hypothyroidism can occur in >10% of cases and hepatic toxicity has been

reported in 75% of patients (Quach et al., 2011). Secondary malignancies have been reported in up to 5% of cases (Weiss et al., 2003).

2.6.7. Recommendations

(69) Although patients frequently present with advanced disease, long-term survival is not uncommon. The probability of inducing acute myelotoxicity, the potential for longer-term secondary neoplasms, and the need to justify administrations of high activity to children and young people emphasise the need for personalised dosimetric planning and verification for all.

2.7. Treatment with radiolabelled peptide receptor

(70) Neuroendocrine tumours express somatostatin receptors. Radiolabelled analogues of somatostatin have been developed for therapeutic purposes including ^{90}Y-DOTATOC ([^{90}Y-DOTA^0,Tyr^3]-octreotide) and ^{177}Lu-DOTATATE ([^{177}Lu-DOTA^0,Tyr^3, Thr^8]-octreotide or [^{177}Lu-DOTA^0,Tyr^3]-octreotate) which target the somatostatin receptor subtype 2. To date, a lack of randomised clinical trials has precluded evidence-based guidelines, although limited guidelines have been produced (Ramage et al., 2012) and a guidance document has been published jointly by the International Atomic Energy Agency (IAEA), EANM, and the Society of Nuclear Medicine and Molecular Imaging based predominantly on expert opinion (Bodei et al., 2013).

(71) The ideal radionuclide has not been established and there are arguments to support both ^{90}Y and ^{177}Lu. ^{90}Y, with a substantially longer range of beta particles, is more able to deposit a uniform distribution of energy at a multi-cellular scale in the event of heterogeneous uptake, whereas it has been argued that this can produce greater kidney toxicity due to irradiation of the cortex (Bodei et al., 2008). ^{177}Lu also has the advantage of photon emissions useful for quantitative imaging for dosimetry, whereas ^{90}Y is often tagged with a tracer level of ^{111}In. The physical half-lives of both radionuclides (64 h and 6.7 days for ^{90}Y and ^{177}Lu, respectively) are compatible with biological retention following uptake. Both ^{177}Lu-DOTATATE and ^{90}Y-DOTATATE are radiolabelled in house, necessitating the usual precautions for the staff at such procedures.

2.7.1. Aim of treatment

(72) Response is variable and the aim of treatment is predominantly palliative. Partial or complete objective responses have been reported in up to 30% of patients; in particular, complete responses have been reported in 26% of patients with gastro-enteropancreatic tumours (Bodei et al., 2013). Treatments are usually administered to adults, although one clinical trial has investigated the potential of ^{177}Lu-DOTATATE treatment of children and young people with neuroblastoma (Gains et al., 2011).

2.7.2. Treatment protocols

(73) Treatment protocols have been standardised with some variations. ^{90}Y-DOTATATE or ^{90}Y-DOTATOC is administered as 3.7 GBq m^{-2} body surface for two cycles or with a fixed activity of 2.78–4.44 GBq for two to four cycles. ^{177}Lu-DOTATATE is commonly administered as a fixed activity of 5.55–7.4 GBq over three to five cycles. The interval between administrations varies from 6 to 12 weeks (Bodei et al., 2013). Patients with compromised renal function are given lower activities. Patients with compromised marrow reserves may require a stem cell harvest for subsequent re-infusion, although haematological toxicity is generally low. Combination therapies of ^{90}Y- and ^{177}Lu-DOTATATE administered alternately are currently under investigation (Kunikowska et al., 2011; Savolainen et al., 2012; Seregni et al., 2014). Dose escalation trials have not established optimal administration protocols.

(74) High levels of somatostatin receptors are observed in children and young people with neuroendocrine tumours, although, with few exceptions, clinical trials exclude this patient population due to an unknown safety profile (Menda et al., 2010; Schmidt et al., 2010; Gains et al., 2011).

2.7.3. Radiation dose to friends and family

(75) Activity is excreted through body fluids, primarily urine and perspiration. Care must therefore be taken when a patient is discharged from hospital, and home circumstances should be taken into account. An individual risk assessment may be required to determine any restrictions on close contact with friends and family when the patient returns home.

2.7.4. Radiation dose to staff

(76) For beta-emitting radionuclides, including ^{90}Y and ^{177}Lu, particular attention should be given to protect staff who prepare and handle the radiopharmaceuticals. Shielded syringes should be used during the intravenous administration of radiopharmaceuticals as necessary to ensure that extremity doses are maintained below occupational dose limits. Equivalent doses to the finger tips from preparation and administration are typically in the range of 5–10 mSv from single administrations when protection is optimised, but can be >100 mSv if precautions are inadequate. Monitoring the equivalent dose to the finger tips using finger stall dosimeters for the main fingers carrying out manipulations is advised for radiological protection to give a reliable indication of finger dose (Cremonesi et al., 2006b; ICRP, 2008; Grassi et al., 2009; Vanhavere et al., 2012).

2.7.5. Patient organ dosimetry

(77) Internal dosimetry is employed routinely in only a minority of centres, and may be applied to tumours and to organs at risk including the kidneys and liver.

Absorbed doses per administered activity from ^{90}Y-DOTATATE to active marrow, kidneys, and liver have been reported as 0.03–0.17 Gy GBq^{-1}, 1.71–2.73 Gy GBq^{-1}, and 0.27–0.92 Gy GBq^{-1}, respectively (Cremonesi et al., 2006a, 2010; Bodei et al., 2008). Absorbed doses per administered activity from ^{177}Lu-DOTATATE to active marrow, kidneys, and liver have been reported as 0.02–0.07 Gy GBq^{-1}, 0.32–1.67 Gy GBq^{-1}, and 0.05–0.21 Gy GBq^{-1}, respectively. Although correlations between absorbed dose and effect have not been an endpoint of any clinical trial to date, there is increasing evidence of such correlations covering both response (Pauwels et al., 2005; Ilan et al., 2015) and toxicity (Barone et al., 2005; Walrand et al., 2011; Strigari et al., 2014). Absorbed dose varies significantly from one patient to another (Hindorf et al., 2007; Sundlöv et al., 2017).

2.7.6. Risks to patients

(78) As with all therapeutic procedures, pregnancy/breast feeding is a contraindication, and patients should avoid conception. Excretion is predominantly urinary and, hence, amino acids are routinely co-administered to protect the kidneys. Kidney toxicity is observed in some patients (Barone et al., 2005; Imhof et al., 2011), and a biologically effective dose (BED) not to exceed 28 Gy (see Section 4.7) has been recommended for patients with higher risk factors treated with ^{90}Y-DOTATATE (Bodei et al., 2008). Grade 3–4 myelotoxicity is observed in up to 10–13% of patients, and cases of myelodysplastic syndrome or overt acute myelogenous leukaemia have been reported (Valkema et al., 2002; Barone et al., 2005; Kwekkeboom et al., 2005; Bushnell et al., 2010; Strosberg et al., 2017).

2.7.7. Recommendations

(79) Data show evidence for acute toxicity primarily to the kidneys and bone marrow. The variation in absorbed doses delivered to tumours and the potential for acute-radiation-induced nephrotoxicity and myelosuppression mean that prospective patient-specific organ and tissue dosimetry should be performed for all patients. The prospect of personalised treatments based on carefully designed dosimetric protocols is quite feasible. There is some evidence that biological parameters such as BED can be of benefit to estimate risks of toxicity to organs at risk, and these should be investigated further (Barone et al., 2005; Wessels et al., 2008).

2.8. Radioimmunotherapy

(80) Radioimmunotherapy involves radiolabelled antibodies that target and bind to tumour-specific antigens, and deliver enhanced therapeutic radiation to neoplasms (Barbet et al., 2012). Antibodies may be mouse monoclonal antibodies or, in many cases, human/mouse chimeric or humanised antibodies that are obtained by genetic engineering technologies in order to reduce immunogenicity in humans. Common

radionuclides include beta emitters such as ^{131}I, ^{90}Y, ^{186}Re, and ^{153}Sm, and alpha emitters such as ^{225}Ac and ^{213}Bi (Sgouros et al., 2010; Larson et al., 2015).

(81) Agents approved by health authorities for general use include ^{131}I-tositumomab and ^{90}Y-ibritumomab tiuxetan (Goldsmith, 2010). Both are directed to CD20-positive, relapsed or refractory, low-grade or follicular B-cell non-Hodgkin's lymphoma. Both agents have a high response rate, with many patients experiencing long-term cancer-free survival. ^{90}Y-ibritumomab tiuxetan is effectively applied to patients with previously untreated lymphoma who achieve a partial or complete response to first-line chemotherapy (Chatal et al., 2008). A number of radioimmunotherapy agents are currently in development or in early phase trials, targeting other indications including neuroblastoma (Kramer et al., 2007), leukaemia (Miederer et al., 2004), and ovarian carcinoma (Andersson et al., 2009).

(82) To date, no radioimmunotherapeutic agent has proved to be effective in achieving sufficiently high absorbed dose to treat solid cancers. Research continues to investigate the efficacy of radioimmunotherapy, with efforts to improve therapeutic ratios with pretargeting (Goldenberg et al., 2012) and increased use of alpha emitters.

2.8.1. Aim of treatment

(83) As radioimmunotherapy encompasses a range of procedures, the aim of treatment is generally to eradicate tumour tissues that express tumour-associated antigens.

2.8.2. Treatment protocols

(84) Treatment regimens vary widely for radioimmunotherapeutic procedures. ^{90}Y-ibritumomab tiuxetan therapy has well-established treatment protocols. Rituximab at $250\,mg\,m^{-2}$ is infused over 4 h, followed by an infusion per body weight of $14.8\,MBq\,kg^{-1}$ of ^{90}Y-ibritumomab tiuxetan, not exceeding 1184 MBq. In some countries and regions, prior to ^{90}Y-ibritumomab tiuxetan therapy, imaging with ^{111}In-ibritumomab tiuxetan is performed according to a therapeutic protocol implemented to verify the expected biodistribution and exclude patients who show an altered biodistribution, such as rapid clearance from the blood pool, with prominent liver, spleen, or marrow uptake (Hanaoka et al., 2015).

2.8.3. Radiation dose to friends and family

(85) Exposure of friends and family is dependent on the radionuclide administered, and the relevant procedures should be followed accordingly. Activity is excreted through body fluids, primarily urine and perspiration. Care must therefore be taken when a patient is discharged, and home circumstances should be taken into account.

2.8.4. Radiation dose to staff

(86) Careful attention should be taken for handling of beta-emitting radiopharmaceuticals, similar to the previous section. In particular, attention should be paid to finger equivalent dose for preparation of ^{90}Y-ibritumomab tiuxetan because high radiation dose has been reported (ICRP, 2008; Vanhavere et al., 2012).

2.8.5. Patient organ dosimetry

(87) A large number of dosimetric studies have been performed related to radioimmunotherapeutic procedures (Cremonesi et al., 2007; Fisher et al., 2009). In Phase III trials of ^{90}Y-ibritumomab tiuxetan, the median estimated radiation absorbed doses were 0.71 and 14.84 Gy to active bone marrow and tumour, respectively (Wiseman et al., 2001). In radioimmunotherapy, radiation dose to organs at risk, including the liver, lungs, intestine, and kidneys, in relation to given radiolabelled antibodies should be evaluated carefully using clinical tests and imaging modalities.

2.8.6. Risks to patients

(88) In cases of radiolabelled antibodies such as ^{131}I-tositumomab and ^{90}Y-ibritumomab tiexetan, acute toxicity is primarily haematologic, causing thrombocytopenia and leukocytopenia. Marrow toxicity needs careful management in patients with fewer bone marrow reserves due to prior repeated chemotherapies. Immunogenic response against the antibody is also a potential concern and should be monitored carefully. As with all therapeutic procedures, pregnancy and breast feeding are contraindicated, and patients should avoid conception until the radioactivity has cleared.

2.8.7. Recommendations

(89) Individual absorbed dose estimates must be performed for treatment planning and postadministration verification of dosimetry on an individualised basis. ^{111}In is commonly used as an imaging surrogate for ^{90}Y.

2.8.8. Emerging technologies in radioimmunotherapy

(90) A number of new radiotherapeutics are currently under development, some of which have already reached the stages of clinical studies to evaluate safety and efficacy in humans. Examples of new methods that have recently attracted worldwide attention include, but are not limited to, targeting prostate-specific membrane antigens (PSMA) for treating prostate cancer, and radioimmunotherapy with alpha emitters for haematological malignancies such as anti-CD33 antibody labelled with ^{213}Bi or ^{225}Ac for acute myeloid leukaemia (Jurcic and Rosenblat, 2014). Another approach to radiopharmaceutical therapy involves pretargeting techniques, which

can enhance tumour to normal tissue accumulation ratios, and therefore the anti-tumour effect of treatment. Pretargeting techniques, which are more complex than conventional techniques, might require more tailored considerations in safe and efficacious usage. Radiological protection standards should be established for these new methods, although it will take some time until sufficient data on radiation doses and risks, as well as on patient care, are accumulated in clinical studies.

2.8.8.1. Therapy with anti-PSMA radiopharmaceuticals

(91) PSMA is overexpressed in prostate cancer, especially in dedifferentiated or castration-resistant cases. Radiolabelled anti-PSMA constructs for imaging that target PSMA have recently been the subject of a number of studies showing high diagnostic accuracy in detecting primary tumours, recurrence, and metastases with good detection rates. The PSMA expression in prostate cancer also provides an approach for new radiopharmaceuticals for therapy. Some anti-PSMA radioimmu-noconjugates have advantages of high affinity that produce good tumour to normal tissue contrast, as well as the ability to be labelled with ^{68}Ga for imaging and ^{177}Lu for therapy. Several studies have reported promising results for response rates and a favourable safety profile after therapy with ^{177}Lu-PSMA-617 in patients with meta-static castration-resistant prostate cancer (Rahbar et al., 2017). Another application of anti-PSMA constructs for radiopharmaceutical therapy has been reported as an initial experience with targeted ^{225}Ac-PSMA-617 alpha therapy in a limited number of patients (Kratochwil et al., 2016). Such alpha-emitter-labelled anti-PSMA con-structs may have good potential for treatment of prostate cancer.

2.8.8.2. Radioimmunotherapy with alpha emitters

(92) As alpha particles have a relatively short range and a high linear energy transfer, radioimmunotherapy with alpha emitters offers the potential for efficient tumour cell killing while sparing surrounding normal cells (Jurcic and Rosenblat, 2014). To date, clinical studies of alpha-particle immunotherapy for acute myeloid leukaemia have focused on the myeloid cell surface antigen CD33 as a target using monoclonal antibodies. Clinical studies have demonstrated safety, feasibility, and anti-leukaemic effects of ^{213}Bi-labelled anti-CD33 antibodies. A conjugate to ^{225}Ac (physical half-life of 10 days) was developed because the use of ^{213}Bi is limited by its short half-life of 46 min (Jurcic and Rosenblat, 2014).

2.8.8.3. Pretargeting techniques

(93) Pretargeting strategies have been introduced to enhance specific tumour uptake in radionuclide therapy. An example of pretargeting techniques is radio-immunotherapy in which the antibody is not labelled but is used to provide binding

sites to low-molecular-weight radioactivity vectors. Such techniques have been shown to increase tumour to non-target uptake ratios, and anti-tumour efficacy has been demonstrated in clinical studies (Chatal et al., 1995; Kraeber-Bodere et al., 2006). Another example of pretargeting involves affibody (small proteins engineered to bind to a high number of target proteins) molecule-based peptide-nucleic-acid-mediated pretargeting, which increased radionuclide uptake in tumours in preclinical studies (Honarvar et al., 2016).

2.9. Intra-arterial treatment of hepatocellular carcinoma and liver metastases by selective internal radiation therapy (SIRT)

(94) Hepatocellular carcinoma and liver metastases may be treated by direct infusion of a radiotherapeutic substance into the hepatic artery, and selective catheterisation of the hepatic artery branches that supply the tumours. Liver tumours preferentially take their blood supply from the hepatic artery, while normal liver is predominantly fed by the portal vein. In recent years, two commercial products, both radiolabelled with ^{90}Y, have become the mainstay for these treatments: glass microspheres (Therasphere, BTG Plc, Ontario, Canada) and resin microspheres (SIR-Spheres, SIRTex Medical Limited, Sydney, Australia). These products have similar properties but differ in terms of the size of the particles and the concentration of activity on each sphere (Giammarile et al., 2011). ^{166}Ho microspheres are currently under development (Smits et al., 2012). Microsphere brachytherapy involves angiography and embolisation of branches not supplying a tumour before microspheres are injected.

(95) Microsphere brachytherapy offers the potential to deliver high absorbed doses to small and large liver lesions with precision targeting. Potential disadvantages include a relatively invasive procedure and the likely irradiation of normal tissue (primarily normal liver tissue, lungs, and intestines) with potentially fatal implications (Giammarile et al., 2011).

2.9.1. Aim of treatment

(96) The primary aim of treatment is curative therapy; some complete responses and long remissions have been reported.

2.9.2. Treatment protocols

(97) A number of formulae are employed to determine the level of activity to administer. Current treatment protocols for microspheres, including monocompartmental and partition models, are based on levels of activity administered or activity per body surface area. The major risk pertains to undesirable or inadvertent placement of microspheres in normal liver. Lung shunting is a risk; therefore, a pretherapy whole-body ^{99m}Tc-MAA (macro-aggregated albumin) scan is performed and

administered activities are modified accordingly. If the lung shunt is too great, administration of ^{90}Y microspheres is contraindicated. The potential for redistribution to the bowel, stomach, or pancreas must also be considered (Lambert et al., 2010). Post-therapy scanning of the liver is usually performed to ensure uptake. ^{90}Y bremsstrahlung imaging is sometimes used, although in recent years, PET imaging has been developed following successful investigation into the low positron yield of ^{90}Y, which is sufficient for the high concentrations of activity localised in tumour and normal liver (Lhommel et al., 2010).

2.9.3. Radiation dose to friends and family

(98) ^{90}Y is a pure beta emitter, and bremsstrahlung emitted from a treated patient is not sufficient to represent a radiation hazard to friends and family after therapy.

2.9.4. Radiation dose to staff

(99) ^{90}Y microspheres are medical devices rather than radiopharmaceutical agents. The most important radiation safety concern is proper administration to patients and contamination control in the healthcare setting prior to administration. Microspheres should be treated as unsealed sources of radiation, and standard precautions must be taken for care and imaging.

2.9.5. Patient organ dosimetry

(100) Dosimetry is performed to guide treatment. Methods based on calculations of the absorbed doses delivered to tumours and normal liver (partition or multi-compartmental modelling) have been developed although there are, as yet, few published standard methodologies (Cremonesi et al., 2014) and gross assumptions are frequently made. For example, the dosimetric method developed for glass spheres is used to calculate the mean absorbed doses to the whole liver, inclusive of any tumour involvement. In recent years, post-therapy imaging and dosimetry have been developed using the low-frequency positron emissions from ^{90}Y that enable the use of PET for both imaging and dosimetry (Willowson et al., 2015).

2.9.6. Risks to patients

(101) Microspheres are designated as medical brachytherapy devices. Irradiation of normal liver parenchyma, either from localisation within the liver or from cross-irradiation from localisation in liver tumours, is a significant risk factor. Radiation-induced liver disease has not been clearly defined to date. There is evidence that an initial state of cirrhosis affects the tolerability to radioembolisation (Chiesa et al., 2011). Delivery of radiation to the pancreas will cause abdominal pain, acute pancreatitis, or peptic ulceration. Lung shunting occurs when administered activity

passes into the pulmonary circulation, and may result in radiation pneumonitis. Inadvertent delivery to the gall bladder may result in cholecystitis. Shunting to the lungs, gastrointestinal tract, or pancreas will vary from one procedure to the next, and therefore absorbed dose limiting toxicity is not possible to predict without pre-therapy biodistribution scanning. Treatment verification is essential following therapy administration as infusion locations may not be guaranteed, and may be modified from the pretherapy work-up. As with all therapeutic procedures, pregnancy/breast feeding is a contraindication, and patients should avoid conception.

2.9.7. Recommendations

(102) The potential to induce severe toxicity or even to cause death, combined with the probability of undertreating many patients, necessitates the use of personalised dosimetry for treatment planning. The lack of certainty regarding the ability of the pretherapy ^{99m}Tc-MAA imaging study to predict the absorbed dose distribution delivered at therapy, exacerbated by the possibility of administering the therapy to a different location from that used for the tracer study, renders post-treatment verification essential if the effect of treatment is to be understood.

2.10. Treatment of arthritis (radionuclide synovectomy)

(103) The administration of radiopharmaceuticals for the treatment of rheumatoid or osteoarthritis has been used for over 40 years (Ansell et al., 1963), and has become well established and widely used; it is also used for treatment of haemophilic synovitis. Synovectomy is a well-tolerated option with significant advantages over surgery and intra-articular administrations of steroids or chemical synovectomy.

(104) Following initial administrations with ^{198}Au, radionuclides with higher beta-particle energies and longer path length are now commonly used, including ^{90}Y and ^{32}P colloid for larger joints such as the knee, ^{186}Re colloid for smaller joints including the elbows and ankle, and ^{169}Er-citrate for the metatarsophalangeal joints (Knut, 2015).

2.10.1. Aim of treatment

(105) The aim of radiosynovectomy is to reduce inflammation and swelling, and to provide pain relief. Reduction of knee joint swelling has been seen in >40% of patients and pain relief in 88%. Wrist, elbow, shoulder, ankle, and hip joints have shown significant improvement, and restoration of normal function and long-term pain relief has been achieved in approximately 70% of small finger joints. In haemophilic arthropathies, complete cessation of bleeding has been seen in 60% of patients and improved mobility in 75% (Das, 2007).

2.10.2. Treatment protocols

(106) Radiopharmaceuticals for synovectomy can be administered at intervals, typically 3 months apart, following a successful first treatment. Repeated treatments are more effective than single treatments with higher activity. Current levels of activity administered have a small evidence base and are derived empirically (Johnson et al., 1995).

2.10.3. Radiation dose to friends and family

(107) Dose to friends and family is not a concern for radiation synovectomy.

2.10.4. Radiation dose to staff

(108) Procedures are standardised as for diagnostic administrations, and precautions must be undertaken, with the use of syringe shields where necessary. Exposures of radiopharmacists and nurses have been found to be within limits for occupationally exposed staff, and doses to therapists working in centres with high numbers of patients have also been reported to be low (Lancelot et al., 2008).

2.10.5. Patient dosimetry

(109) Absorbed dose calculations were addressed previously (Bowring and Keeling, 1978) when it was considered that the challenges of uptake and target localisation, quantification of activity, and monitoring of retention were scientifically and logistically prohibitive. A comprehensive approach to dosimetry for radiosynovectomy ideally requires a Monte Carlo approach which enables the production of depth dose profiles for any given radionuclide (Johnson et al., 1995).

2.10.6. Risks to patients

(110) The limited range of intra-articular injected radionuclides, while in situ, ensures few adverse tissue reactions by irradiation of adjacent tissues. Reported side effects are rare and are generally related to the administration procedure (comprising joint inflammation and skin necrosis from extra-articular administrations). The radiation exposure of the whole body of patients is very low for beta-emitting radionuclides because of the limited range of beta emissions (10 mm for ^{90}Y and $\leq$1 mm for ^{169}Er). No genotoxic effects were found in peripheral blood following administration of ^{90}Y-citrate in children with haemophilic synovitis (Klett et al., 1999; Turkmen et al., 2007). Absorbed doses delivered to the lymph nodes, liver, spleen, and whole body have been calculated as 619 (154–1644) mGy, 62 (15–165) mGy, 62 (15–165) mGy, and 37 (9–99) mGy, respectively, and leakage rates from sequential imaging are reported to be <2% (Klett et al., 1999). In a large Canadian study of patients receiving radiosynovectomy with ^{90}Y, no increase in

the incidence of cancer was observed in 2412 adult patients with a variety of under-lying conditions, although the study concluded that further investigation was needed for procedures for younger patients (Infante-Rivard et al., 2012). As with all ther-apeutic procedures, pregnancy/breast feeding is a contraindication, and patients should avoid conception.

2.10.7. Recommendations

(111) It is important to verify the intra-articular position of the needle before the patient is administered with the treatment radionuclide. Leakage of particulates has been demonstrated to be low in animal models with sequential gamma camera imaging, and is expected to be low in humans (Noble et al., 1983). However, studies are needed to confirm this assumption.

3. BIOKINETIC DATA COLLECTION

3.1. Whole-body activity

(112) Although radionuclides for therapy need to have short range emissions to focus dose delivery within target tissues, whole-body monitoring of organ and tissue uptake and retention rely on the radionuclide also having penetrating photon emissions. For radionuclides with penetrating photon or bremsstrahlung emissions, the activity in the whole body can be measured with a detector at a distance >2 m. The first data point is taken before the patient micturates so that this value can be used for normalising the data set to 100%. All subsequent measurements must be performed in the same geometry. This procedure is correct only if the sensitivity of the probe is independent of the distribution of activity in the patient. This is normally the case, if the photons scattered by the patient are eliminated by spectroscopic measurements that only include the photo peak of the radionuclide in question (Lassmann et al., 2008).

(113) The determination of activity of the whole body can also be performed by repeated whole-body scans with a gamma camera. Post therapeutically, it has to be ascertained that the dead time correction of the camera is set up properly (Hänscheid et al., 2006; Lassmann et al., 2008).

3.2. Activity in the blood

(114) This method is typically applied for determining the absorbed dose to blood (Lassmann et al., 2008; Hänscheid et al., 2009) or bone marrow (Hindorf et al., 2010). The kinetics of activity in blood are typically measured by serial sampling of heparinised blood and subsequent measurement in a calibrated well counter. Dependent on the biokinetics of the compound considered, at least one blood sample needs to be withdrawn at a later stage (e.g. at or beyond 96 h post injection) (Lassmann et al., 2008).

3.3. Organ and tumour activity

3.3.1. Quantitative imaging

(115) Quantitatively accurate imaging is required for treatment planning and evaluation of radiopharmaceutical therapy. Over the past years, progress has been made in development of methods for accurate quantification of nuclear medicine images. However, extension of these methods into most clinics has been slow.

(116) Achieving quantification requires appropriate equipment, software, and human resources. The level of these requirements depends on the specific

requirement for quantitative imaging. For example, quantifying activity in a tumour in the lungs requires more sophisticated resources than quantifying whole-body activity.

(117) While, in general, multiple uses of sophisticated imaging devices enable better determination of the biokinetics of a radiopharmaceutical, this benefit must be weighed against what is practically achievable. On the one hand, a few probe measurements could provide valuable insights into whole-body retention in the individual patient. Multiple SPECT/computed tomography (CT) or PET/CT sessions can be helpful for determining the biokinetics of novel therapeutic radiopharmaceuticals.

(118) The type and number of imaging sessions needed for a particular patient undergoing radiopharmaceutical therapy should be optimised. Consideration should include availability of personnel and equipment, financial and logistical costs, expected accuracy of quantification, radiation dose to imaging technologists, and any possible patient discomfort.

(119) This section provides a brief overview of the technology involved in quantitatively accurate imaging. More thorough descriptions such as IAEA Human Health Reports No. 9 can be consulted for more details (IAEA, 2014b).

3.3.2. Planar imaging

(120) Today, planar imaging with a gamma camera for dosimetric purposes is useful for determining organ uptake and clearance biokinetics, and individual organ overlap must be assessed accurately, taking into account attenuation, scatter, and background correction (Siegel et al., 1999).

(121) Planar images are most commonly used with dual-head cameras (Siegel et al., 1999; Glatting et al., 2005). For opposite scintillation detectors, the pixel-wise geometric mean of the counts in a source-organ region of interest represents a first-order approximation for activity in the corresponding pixel (conjugate view method). The dependency of the measured count-rate I_{PQ} (counts s^{-1}) on activity A_{PQ} (MBq) of a point source PQ is:

$$I_{PQ} = C \cdot A_{PQ} \cdot e^{-\mu_e x} \qquad (3.1)$$

where C is the calibration coefficient (counts MBq^{-1} s^{-1}) of the camera head, μ_e (cm^{-1}) is the effective linear attenuation coefficient, and x (cm) is the depth of the point source in the body. The geometric mean of the count rates G (counts s^{-1}) for two opposite camera heads and the thickness of the body D (cm) is calculated as:

$$G = \sqrt{I_a \cdot I_p} = A_{PQ} \cdot C \cdot \sqrt{e^{-\mu_e x} \cdot e^{-\mu_e (D-x)}} = A_{PQ} \cdot C \cdot e^{-\mu_e D/2} \qquad (3.2)$$

where I_a and I_p are the measured anterior and posterior count rates, and $C = \sqrt{C_a \cdot C_p}$ is the calibration factor for the geometric mean of both camera heads. Solving Eq. (3.2) for the unknown activity A_{PQ} results in:

$$A_{PQ} = \frac{\sqrt{I_a \cdot I_p}}{C} \, e^{\mu_e D/2} \tag{3.3}$$

(122) Thus, the thickness of the investigated object or patient and linear attenuation coefficient are required for determining the activity of a point source when using two opposite camera heads. This equation is valid when the gamma detector sensitivity is not dependent on the distance from the source. As this is only approximately true, the error can be more than 100% depending on the radionuclide, the energy window, and the collimator in comparison with the mid-position of the point source (Glatting and Lassmann, 2007).

3.3.3. SPECT/CT

(123) To measure activity in the accumulating organs and tumours using imaging techniques, quantification by means of SPECT/CT for at least one data point is state of the art. Due to the inclusion of scattering and attenuation correction, accuracies >10% are achievable in phantom measurements (Dewaraja et al., 2012, 2013).

(124) The calibration of imaging systems is essential for patient-specific dosimetry in nuclear medicine therapy, but standardisation methods are not commonly followed. Appropriate calibration sources may not be readily available for radionuclides which are used pretherapeutically as a substitute for ^{90}Y (e.g. ^{111}In), or for short-lived radionuclides used therapeutically (e.g. ^{131}I, ^{177}Lu). Therefore, calibration usually relies on fillable calibration phantoms using a known activity of the radionuclide that will be administered.

(125) For calibrating and determining the optimal parameters for quantifying SPECT/CT, a large calibration source in air and in water filled with the radioactive substances should be scanned and reconstructed in order to obtain the appropriate values. For the best quantification, the following conditions should be met (Dewaraja et al., 2012, 2013; Fernández Tomás et al., 2012; Zimmerman et al., 2017).

- A finer angular grid with reduced scanning times is better than a coarse grid (Dewaraja et al., 2012).
- Committee on Medical Internal Radiation Dose (MIRD) Pamphlet 26 (Ljungberg et al., 2016) states that iterative methods require a certain number of updates before reaching an acceptable image quality. MIRD Pamphlet 23 (Dewaraja et al., 2012) defines the convergence as the point when 90% recovery has been reached, representing high reconstruction accuracy. More complex reconstruction problems (having more corrections in the algorithm) require more iterations to reach convergence. Reconstruction parameters may be

optimised using data from phantom studies and simulations, and also sample patient data with representative activity distributions and counting statistics. Due to the limited spatial resolution of SPECT/CT, when using the CT volume or a fixed threshold for volume-of-interest drawing, it is advisable to implement corrections for the partial-volume effect. For an empirical correction of the spill-out of the counts, the volume of interest may be increased to account for the spatial resolution of the SPECT/CT system in comparison with the volume measured by CT.

- For ^{111}In and ^{177}Lu, there is no difference in accuracy regardless of whether one or two photo peaks are chosen, provided that the energy windows for the photo peaks and the adjacent scatter windows are chosen correctly. For ^{177}Lu, however, care has to be taken that, for an incorrect window setting of the scatter window for the 113-keV peak, the quantification might show an error >10% (Ljungberg et al., 2016).

(126) In principle, the required organ volumes can be obtained from tomographic emission measurements. The accuracy of these methods, however, especially in smaller structures, is limited due to their relatively poor spatial resolution. In addition, motion artefacts can mask the true organ volume. Therefore, it seems useful to use high-resolution anatomical procedures such as CT scans or magnetic resonance imaging to determine organ and tumour volumes.

3.3.4. PET/CT

(127) The role of PET/CT for therapeutic radiopharmaceuticals has mainly focused on using positron-emitting surrogates of the therapeutic radionuclides, such as [124]I for ^{131}I, and [86]Y for ^{90}Y treatments.

(128) The applicability of quantitative PET/CT imaging of ^{90}Y has, however, been demonstrated for selective internal radiation therapy (Carlier et al., 2015) and other ^{90}Y radiopharmaceuticals. A multi-centre comparison of quantitative ^{90}Y PET/CT for dosimetric purposes after radioembolisation with resin microspheres showed that the current generation time-of-flight scanners can consistently reconstruct ^{90}Y activity concentrations, but underestimate activity concentrations in small structures (≤37-mm diameter) within background activity due to partial volume effects and constraints of the reconstruction algorithm (Willowson et al., 2015).

3.4. Quantitative protocols

3.4.1. Quantitative imaging protocols

(129) Protocols (or standard operating procedures) ensure consistency of data acquisition and processing. A protocol should describe the steps required to obtain satisfactory clinical data and measurements.

(130) The expertise required for writing protocols differs from that required to implement them, and different personnel may be required. Typically, the protocol should be written by a trained medical physicist and medical staff.

(131) Quality assurance and quality control (QA/QC) tasks should be performed at a specified frequency to ensure that the equipment is operating as intended. The schedule for QA/QC procedures should be specified in the protocol. QA/QC results should be provided systematically along with all the data related to the protocol.

3.4.2. Pharmacokinetics and integration of the time–activity curve

(132) The choice of acquisition times for determining the uptake and retention of activity in an organ or defined region of interest influences the reliability of the quantitative assay (Glatting and Lassmann, 2007). An optimised acquisition time may be calculated by plotting the time–activity data for a source region, and then integrating the area under an appropriate function fit to the data. According to the MIRD Pamphlet 21 nomenclature (Bolch et al., 2009), the integral of a time–activity function is the time-integrated activity in the source region (replacing previous term 'cumulated activity'). The number of data points needed depends on the biokinetics in the respective organ or tissue. As a rule of thumb, one needs at least three data points to correctly fit each exponential term in the function (Siegel et al., 1999). The number of exponential terms depends strongly on the tolerated errors of the fitting process.

(133) Many different mathematical and curve-fitting software packages are commercially available for fitting mathematical functions to plots of time–activity data. These software packages usually provide capability for integrating the best-fit function, and provide relevant statistical parameters for ascertaining goodness of fit (Kletting et al., 2013).

(134) As the number of imaging scans that can be reasonably performed on patients is limited by practical considerations, MIRD Pamphlet 16 (Siegel et al., 1999) recommends five measurements at $T_e/3$, $2T_e/3$, $3T_e/2$, $3T_e$, and $5T_e$, where T_e is the effective half-time in the organ or tissue structure considered.

4. METHODS FOR ABSORBED DOSE CALCULATIONS

(135) The use of radiopharmaceuticals for cancer treatment requires detailed, patient-specific dosimetry for assessments of absorbed dose to normal organs and tumour tissues. In treatment planning, the calculation of absorbed dose to internal organs, tissues, and the whole body is a fundamentally important aspect for successfully achieving clinical objectives. Since radiopharmaceuticals are usually administered systemically or orally, radionuclide therapy necessarily involves delivery of some radiation energy to all normal organs and tissues. The amount of activity administered should be sufficient to treat the neoplasm effectively while minimising any detrimental dose to normal tissues. The principle applied in radiation therapy is to maximise the radiation delivered to cancer without exceeding normal tissue tolerance values. Therefore, the activity that may be safely administered for cancer treatment can be determined by assessing absorbed doses to internal organs, with particular attention given to the most important, toxicity-limiting normal tissues.

(136) Quantitative measurements of organ activity over time, and organ mass, are essential to calculate absorbed doses. In radiopharmaceutical therapy treatment planning and for patient safety, it is usually more important to assess normal organ dose accurately than to assess tumour dose. Nonetheless, tumour dose is a factor needed to determine the therapeutic index, a measure of both safety and efficacy. The therapeutic index is the ratio of the dose to the target region (or tumour) relative to the dose to the limiting normal organ dose (D_{tumour}/D_{normal}).

4.1. Purpose of absorbed dose calculations

(137) Absorbed dose calculations are performed prior to therapy on the basis of measurements made following a trace-labelled diagnostic infusion, or after therapy on the basis of measurements following the administration of treatment. Internal radiation dosimetry serves several fundamental purposes in radiopharmaceutical therapy and radiological protection, including:

- to evaluate the safety and efficacy of a therapeutic agent;
- to provide an information source for discussing anticipated absorbed doses with patients;
- to plan an appropriate treatment for radiopharmaceutical therapy;
- to predict short- and long-term radiation effects or dose-related biological endpoints associated with radiotherapy, and to correlate biological effects with radiation dose;
- to provide a required list of estimated radiation doses to internal organs from radiopharmaceuticals;
- to fulfil legal obligations and demonstrate regulatory compliance; and
- to serve as a component of complete patient medical records.

4.2. Data for absorbed dose calculations

(138) In radiopharmaceutical therapy, the time of intake and the amount of activity administered represent known or established quantities, determined by prescription, based on prior estimates of the radiation dose that will be needed to achieve beneficial therapy outcomes.

(139) The major challenge in radiation dose assessment is accurate assessment of the time course (biokinetics) of radionuclide uptake, retention, and clearance in normal organs and tumour tissues. The pharmacokinetic behaviour of radiolabelled drug products is analysed and determined by direct measurements (nuclear medicine imaging) and direct bioassay (blood and excreta counting, and tissue biopsy counting) (see Section 3). Direct measurements may be supplemented by pharmacokinetic modelling using population parametric values. For treatment planning or postinfusion follow-up, individual patient measurements are more reliable than estimates based on population biokinetic models. Since the biodistribution and metabolic behaviour of radiopharmaceuticals usually vary from one patient to another, patient-specific measurements are needed to determine patient-specific biokinetic parameters.

(140) Direct measurements of organ or tissue radioactivity must account for the geometry and density of the source organ or tissue, organ size and mass, potential overlap, thickness of tissue between the organ and the detector, and the spatial distribution of activity within a tissue. Measurements are corrected for body and detector background, detector dead time, and photon attenuation and scatter that may influence the accuracy of direct counting.

(141) For any radionuclide, the information needed to calculate absorbed dose includes: the total activity administered to the patient and time of administration, the fraction of the administered activity that is taken up by each imageable source organ or tissue, and the time-dependent retention and clearance of activity in each major source organ through complete radiological decay.

(142) In the medical setting, measurements of organ activity may be made using calibrated nuclear medicine systems. These include planar gamma camera (anterior/posterior) imaging, SPECT, PET, and single crystal (sodium iodide or other scintillator) photon detectors. The patient is placed within the field of view for quantitative imaging over the thoracic or abdominal regions; alternatively, the patient may receive a whole-body scan for region-of-interest measurements. The imaging procedure is repeated at predetermined time points according to the protocol, following a baseline (before injection) count and a postinjection image immediately after radiopharmaceutical infusion (near time zero). Markers are used to correctly position the patient for repetitive measurements. The technologist selects regions of interest by outlining the major organs or tissue regions. In addition to all regions of interest, it is important to measure whole-body radioactivity over time to determine residual activity in all other non-source organs and tissues (called the 'remainder').

(143) Instrument counts in selected regions of interest are converted to units of activity (Bq) using radionuclide standards, patient thickness measurements,

background subtraction, attenuation correction, and scatter correction techniques. Such instrument counts require availability of photon emissions for quantitative counting. When it is not possible to determine precise activity concentrations in organs and tissues with time, estimates may be made using biokinetic or pharmacokinetic modelling. The quality of the assessment depends on the validity of the model parameters assumed. Modelling can provide important information where data are lacking, but the models are rarely patient-specific, and potential errors that are introduced should be taken into account.

4.3. Absorbed dose

(144) Absorbed dose is the fundamental radiation quantity that describes energy deposition by ionising radiation in an absorbing medium (ICRU, 2016); absorbed dose applies to all radiation exposures, all types of ionising radiation, any absorbing medium, and all biological targets and geometries. Calculation of absorbed dose from intake of radionuclides requires information about the amount of radioactivity present over time periods through complete decay or clearance, the mass and geometry of the target tissue, and all physical factors governing energy deposition after radionuclide decay (ICRP, 2015a,b).

(145) In radiopharmaceutical therapy, the time of intake and the amount of activity administered represent known or established quantities. The amounts of radioactivity present in organs and tissues after administration may be determined by direct quantitative imaging or by sample measurement and pharmacokinetic modelling. Methods that have been developed for medical internal radiation dosimetry greatly simplify the dose assessment task without compromising on essential details. Nuclear medicine imaging, image rendering, and computational capabilities are evolving to meet the needs for accurate and reliable internal dosimetry. Current methods extend from the whole organ to the cellular and multi-cellular levels, and may be applied to either uniform or non-uniform radionuclide distributions within organs and tissues. Patient-specific methods are preferred over generic model assumptions.

(146) For radionuclide therapy, the relevant dosimetric quantity associated with immediate deterministic effects in radiopharmaceutical therapy is the absorbed dose (in $J\,kg^{-1}$). In its most basic form, the absorbed dose, D, to an organ or tissue is simply the mean energy imparted per unit mass of tissue from all ionising radiation components that contribute energy to the target tissue mass:

$$D = \frac{d\bar{\varepsilon}}{dm} \; Gy \; \left(J \cdot kg^{-1}\right) \qquad (4.1)$$

where D is the quotient of the mean energy (d) imparted to an element of matter by ionising radiation and the mass (dm) of the element.

(147) When applied to radionuclides administered to a living biological system and where the source region is the same as the target region, the general absorbed dose

equation includes a biological retention function to account for radionuclide meta-bolism and clearance, as well as the fraction of energy that is captured or absorbed in the target region:

$$D = \left(\frac{AEY\phi}{m}\right) \int_0^t B(t)\, dt \; \text{Gy} \; \left(\text{J kg}^{-1}\right) \tag{4.2}$$

where D is the mean absorbed dose, A is the activity of the radionuclide (Bq), EY is the total energy emitted (J) by the radionuclide in the organ or tissue (product of particle energy and yield), ϕ is the fraction of that energy that is absorbed in the target region, m is the mass of the target region (kg), and $\int_0^t B(t)\, dt$ is the biological retention of the activity integrated from time $t = 0$ (injection) through complete decay or clearance $(t = \infty)$, or for any specific time period, t (s or h). The mass of the target organ should be determined from medical imaging, but standard model values for organ mass may be used if precise data are not available. Eq. (4.2) rear-ranged is:

$$D = A \int_0^t B(t)\, dt \left(\frac{EY\phi}{m}\right) \text{Gy} \; \left(\text{J kg}^{-1}\right) \tag{4.3}$$

which leads directly to the general form of the MIRD schema shown in Eq. (4.4).

(148) The patient comprises multiple source and target organs or tissues. The absorbed dose to any organ or tissue includes all energy deposition event contribu-tions from: (1) radioactivity contained within the organ (the self-organ dose); and (2) all energy depositions originating from radioactivity contained in all other organs and tissues of the whole body (the cross-organ dose). The mean absorbed dose is calculated by accounting for the physical half-life, biological retention, all radioactive emissions by a given radionuclide, and the individual absorbed frac-tions for all radioactive emissions from that radionuclide for any specified source–target geometry in the human body. The complex geometries represented by the human body for any age, sex, height, weight, variations in organ size, and differ-ences in tissue density (skeleton, soft tissue, lungs), taken together, present formid-able challenges for a comprehensive calculation that can account for all important determinants of ε/m for any specified target region. The dose calculation must account for differences in radionuclide biokinetics (uptake, retention, and clear-ance) unique to each organ or tissue for the radiopharmaceutical of interest, together with factors that may determine unique metabolic rates and health status of individual patients and which render differences in pharmacokinetics from one patient to another.

(149) The MIRD schema (Loevinger and Berman, 1968) was developed to account for all physical, biological, and geometric factors for all energy contributions to absorbed dose for any target tissue from radionuclides in multiple source organs and remainder tissues. Since 1968, the MIRD schema has evolved to accommodate modern anatomical views by CT or magnetic resonance imaging, voxel-level activity

distributions, Monte Carlo energy transport codes, pharmacokinetic compartment models, and radiobiological response parameters.

(150) After administration of a radiopharmaceutical via intravenous injection, the drug product redistributes quickly throughout the organs and tissues of the body, and all organs and tissues receive some radiation dose. However, by definition in the MIRD schema, the source organ or region r_S is defined as any tissue mass, organ, tumour, or the whole body for which data are available to determine a time–activity curve. The target organ or region r_T is defined as any organ or tissue for which an absorbed dose can be calculated.

(151) Using the updated MIRD/ICRP formalism and nomenclature (Bolch et al., 2009; ICRP, 2015b), the mean absorbed dose $D(r_T, \tau)$ to a target tissue r_T over a defined dose-integration period τ (infinity for short-lived radionuclides) following administration of a radioactive material to the medical patient is:

$$D(r_T, \tau) = \sum_{r_S} \int_0^t A(r_s, t) S(r_T \leftarrow r_S, t) dt \ \mathrm{Gy} \ \left(\mathrm{J \ kg^{-1}}\right) \tag{4.4}$$

where the quantity $S(r_T \leftarrow r_S, t)$ is the radionuclide-specific quantity representing the mean absorbed dose rate to target region r_T at time t after administration per activity present in source region r_S (Snyder et al., 1969; Bolch et al., 2009). For a specific radionuclide and for a well-defined geometry representing the source–target pair:

$$S(r_T \leftarrow r_S, t) = \frac{1}{m(r_T, t)} \sum_i E_i Y_i \phi(r_T \leftarrow r_S, E_i, t) = \frac{1}{m(r_T, t)} \sum_i \Delta_i \phi(r_T \leftarrow r_S, E_i, t) \tag{4.5}$$

where E_i and Y_i are the energy and yield (number per nuclear transition), respectively, of each radiation particle or photon i emitted by the radionuclide; Δ_i is their product (or mean energy emitted per nuclear transition); and $\phi(r_T \leftarrow r_S, E_i, t)$ is the absorbed fraction of radiation energy E_i emitted by the source region r_S at time t that is absorbed in target tissue r_T.

(152) If the quantity $A(r_s, t)$ is normalised to a unit administered activity A_0 and is designated as the quantity $a(r_s, t)$, the absorbed dose coefficient $d(r_T, \tau)$ in target tissue r_T is (Bolch et al., 2009):

$$d(r_T, \tau) = \sum_{r_S} \int_0^\tau a(r_s, t) S(r_T \leftarrow r_S, t) dt \ \mathrm{GyBq^{-1}} \tag{4.6}$$

where $a(r_s, t) = A(r_s, t)/A_0$ is the fraction of the administered radioactivity remaining in the source tissue r_S at any time t after infusion. The fraction $a(r_s, t)$ is the quantity that is measured for radiation dosimetry in the patient by region-of-interest quantitative imaging using clinical nuclear medicine instruments.

(153) Eq. (4.4) may be simplified, when time dependence of S is neglected, using the time-independent expression:

$$D(r_T, \tau) = \sum_{rs} \tilde{A}(r_s, \tau)S(r_T \leftarrow r_S) \text{ Gy} \qquad (4.7)$$

where the quantity $\tilde{A}(r_s, \tau)$ represents the time-integrated activity (or total number of nuclear decay transitions) in source region r_s for the dose-integration period τ and where:

$$\tilde{A}(r_s, \tau) = \int_0^\tau A(r_s, t)dt \text{ Bq s} \qquad (4.8)$$

(154) Fully implemented, the MIRD/ICRP formalism represented by Eq. (4.7) accounts for all source regions, all target organs, all source–target geometries, and all radioactive emissions contributing to absorbed dose. Tabulated values of S have been published to simplify internal dose calculations for simple source–target geometries. For all other cases, the specific absorbed fractions for a radionuclide and computational phantom model must be calculated individually using a Monte Carlo nuclear transport code that accounts for individual geometry, tissue compositions, and absorber densities. Dosimetric calculations may be performed with a number of commercially available software packages or software developed in house (Guy et al., 2003; McKay, 2003; Glatting et al., 2005; Stabin et al., 2005). Software used for calculation of organ doses and effective doses by ICRP is available (Andersson et al., 2014; ICRP, 2015a; www.idac-dose.org).

4.4. Time-integrated activity coefficient in a source region

(155) The time-integrated activity coefficient $\tilde{a}(r_s, \tau)$ is the area under the time–activity curve representing the integral quantity $\int_0^\tau a(r_s, t)dt$ in Eq. (4.6). This quantity was previously known as the 'residence time' in earlier MIRD publications; it is equal to the ratio of the time-integrated activity and the total administered activity, A_0:

$$\tilde{a}(r_s, \tau) = \int_0^\tau a(r_s, t)dt = \tilde{A}(r_s, \tau)/A_0 \text{ Bq s Bq}^{-1} \text{ or s} \qquad (4.9)$$

(156) The time-integrated activity coefficient is a common input value for software programmes that implement the MIRD/ICRP schema for absorbed dose calculations. The time-integrated activity coefficient for a source region may be determined by plotting the fraction of administered activity in that source region over time and evaluating the area under the curve. Several measurement data points, depending on

the form of the mathematical function, are needed to establish a time–activity curve best represented by the plotted data (Siegel et al., 1999).

(157) The counts obtained in an organ or tissue region of interest must be converted to units of radioactivity using appropriate measurement methods and calibration standards, including: daily quality assurance, patient positioning, patient thickness measurements, background subtraction, attenuation correction, and scatter correction. In planar imaging, the geometric mean of counts obtained from anterior and posterior views is determined. The fraction of administered activity measured in the source region may be plotted as a function of time after infusion. A mathematical function or time–activity curve should then be fitted to the plotted data using linear least-squares regression analysis. Physical decay is exponential, and biological uptake and clearance usually follow exponential patterns; therefore, an exponential function with one or more terms is usually an appropriate function to represent the plotted data. The fitted function is integrated numerically or analytically to yield the time-integrated activity coefficient.

(158) Alternatively, the time-integrated activity coefficient for a source region may be calculated using dynamic modelling if the pharmacokinetic parameters associated with model compartments (source regions) and their associated transfer coefficients are known or can be determined iteratively. When combined with dosimetric subroutines, and following the general MIRD/ICRP schema, biokinetic models may also be used to calculate radiation absorbed doses to target regions directly.

4.5. Uncertainties in absorbed dose calculations

(159) Uncertainty analyses provide information concerning sources and magnitude of bias (accuracy) and random variation (precision), reflecting the reliability and quality of absorbed dose calculations. Internal dose calculations involve a number of measurements, complex anatomical geometries, and variable biological factors when applied to administered radiopharmaceuticals. Details of measurements and sources of modelling errors should therefore be considered. The EANM guidance document on uncertainty analysis presents a framework to model the major sources of dosimetric uncertainty (Gear et al., 2018). Uncertainty should be recognised, acknowledged, and minimised when possible to improve confidence in the calculated absorbed dose.

(160) The total uncertainty in an estimate of the mean absorbed dose to an organ or tissue from a therapeutic radiopharmaceutical administered to a patient reflects different sources of uncertainty: (1) measurement uncertainties associated with quantitative imaging methods used to determine absolute activities in major source regions; (2) uncertainties in estimating integrated activity in organs/tissues; and (3) the application of mathematical phantoms or standard reference models used to represent the anatomical organ geometries of live subjects.

(161) With modern activity measurement instruments (dose calibrators), administered activities may be known to be accurate within a few percent. Differences between planned and actual administered activity are only minor contributors to the total uncertainty if regular quality control is performed (IAEA, 2006a). Uncertainties associated with variances in assumed mass of the target organ may be minimised with use of patient CT and three-dimensional volumetric reconstructions.

(162) Variations in estimated time-integrated activities for major source organs arise from inherent difficulties in measuring and quantifying organ uptake, retention, and redistribution of the radiopharmaceutical in tissues (Norrgren et al., 2003; Jönsson et al., 2005). Uncertainties associated with the shape of the time–activity curve may be minimised by obtaining sufficient data points to establish the time–activity function and optimise statistical fitting to the data. The most important data points are the initial organ uptake near time zero after administration or completion of the infusion, and the last time point that weighs heavily towards helping one to determine the slope of the long-term retention. Typically, a minimum of four or five data points are needed at properly spaced collection times to minimise uncertainty associated with area-under-curve analyses.

(163) Variations in estimates of photon cross-organ contributions to a source region dose, dependent on assumed distances between the source and target organs, contribute to uncertainties in tabulated S values. Physical data, such as the radionuclide emission energies and yields applicable to absorbed fraction calculations for target organs, are well characterised and do not contribute significantly to overall uncertainty.

(164) Experimental measurement validation of calculated absorbed doses using reference anthropomorphic phantoms and mathematical models have indicated agreement within 20–60%, depending on the degree to which subjects compare with the body size and shape assumed in the calculations (Roedler, 1980).

4.6. Biologically effective dose (BED)

(165) When an absorbed dose is delivered by low-linear energy transfer radiation at a low absorbed dose rate, the radiobiological effects are believed to decrease compared with those obtained for the same absorbed dose delivered with a high dose rate. The decrease is associated with repair of DNA damage during irradiation, depending on the tissue repair capacity and the rate of repair in relation to the time of radiation delivery. Other time-dependent factors that may modify the cellular response include proliferation (repopulation), redistribution in the cell cycle, and re-oxygenation (Joiner and van der Kogel, 2009).

(166) In radiopharmaceutical therapy, the absorbed dose rate in an organ or tissue is governed by the radiopharmaceutical uptake and retention in the organ itself and in surrounding organs, combined with the radionuclide physical half-life. The radiation delivery can extend over long time periods (days or even weeks) (Gleisner et al.,

2015). The absorbed dose rate varies over time, and the mean absorbed dose rate is considerably lower than in most other forms of radiotherapy. Spatial heterogeneities also influence response, such as those governed by the molecular mechanisms for radiopharmaceutical accumulation and the range of the particles that are emitted during radioactive decay.

(167) Applications of the linear-quadratic radiobiological model were described previously for radiopharmaceutical therapy (Millar, 1991; Howell et al., 1994; Dale, 1996) to estimate the fraction of cells surviving the irradiation, SF, as follows:

$$SF = \mathrm{e}^{-\left(\alpha D + G(T)\beta D^2\right)} \tag{4.10}$$

where D is the absorbed dose delivered from the start of irradiation until time T, and α and β are radiobiological parameters that characterise the shape of the cell survival curve.

(168) The first term in the exponent (linear in D) dominates the cell-survival curve at low absorbed doses; the first term may be associated with lethal DNA damage induced by single-particle tracks (Dale, 1996). The second, a quadratic term, describes the increasingly downward curvature for SF at higher absorbed doses; it has been interpreted as the effects from pairwise interaction of sublethal lesions induced by two particle tracks. The function G, called the 'Lea-Catcheside factor', acts as a damping of the second term, and is deduced from the perspective that there is a probability that the first sublethal DNA lesion is repaired before the second is induced. G is formally defined as (Lea and Catcheside, 1942; Kellerer and Rossi, 1974):

$$G(T) = \frac{2}{D^2} \int_0^T R(t)\left[\int_0^t R(w)\varphi(t - w)\mathrm{d}w\right]\mathrm{d}t \tag{4.11}$$

where $R(t)$ is the absorbed dose rate as a function of time. The function $\varphi(t)$ describes the loss of sublethal lesions due to repair, and is often assumed to be a single-phase process with a repair half-time T_{rep} and rate constant $\mu = \ln(2)/T_{\mathrm{rep}}$, such that:

$$\varphi(t) = e^{-\mu t} \tag{4.12}$$

although multi-phase repair processes have also been reported (Joiner and van der Kogel, 2009). The function $G(T)$ takes values between 0 and 1 depending on the rate of repair in relation to the rate of cell-lesion induction, in turn proportional to the absorbed dose rate.

(169) For most radionuclide therapies, irradiation continues until the radionuclide has decayed or been excreted. For an absorbed dose rate function described by an

effective decay constant, λ, combined with Eq. (4.12) and after integration of Eq. (4.11) to infinity, $G(T)$ takes the form:

$$\lim_{T \to \infty} G(T) = \frac{\lambda}{\lambda + \mu} \qquad (4.13)$$

Analytic solution of Eq. (4.11) for more complicated absorbed dose rate patterns or repair functions is challenging; the integral within brackets in Eq. (4.11) can be described as a convolution (Gustafsson et al., 2013a). This formulation allows for numerical implementation, which opens for application of more complex absorbed dose rate functions and repair functions other than mono-exponential functions (Gustafsson et al., 2013b).

(170) BED is a concept within the framework of the linear-quadratic model (Barendsen, 1982; Fowler, 1989; Dale, 1996; Joiner and van der Kogel, 2009). The concept of BED relies on the idea of equieffective treatments [i.e. treatments that produce the same probability of inducing a specific clinical (biological) endpoint] (Bentzen et al., 2012). The main use of BED is found in external-beam radiotherapy and brachytherapy, where it is a clinically accepted method for converting between different fractionation schemes and absorbed dose rate patterns. In radiopharmaceutical therapy, its usefulness for describing clinically observed effects has been demonstrated (Barone et al., 2005; Wessels et al., 2008; Strigari et al., 2010). Barone et al. (2005) found that kidney toxicity correlated better with BED than with absorbed dose, and in MIRD Pamphlet No. 20 (Wessels et al., 2008), the relationship between BED and the incidence of renal complications was comparable with that obtained for external-beam radiotherapy. Strigari et al. (2010) described a relationship between BED and the normal tissue complication probability of liver.

(171) For organs and tissue, the biologic effect may be expressed with a functional form that is equivalent to the logarithm of cell killing in Eq. (4.10): $\ln(S)$. BED is then calculated according to:

$$\text{BED} = D + \frac{G(T)}{\alpha/\beta} D^2 = D\left(1 + \frac{G(T) \cdot D}{\alpha/\beta}\right) = D \cdot RE \qquad (4.14)$$

where the α/β value is characteristic for the organ or tissue and the endpoint that is an observed effect. The formulation of BED as the product of D and relative effectiveness (RE) has been given by Barendsen (1982) and Dale (1996). In their notation, RE is the ratio of absorbed doses required to yield a given equieffect, where BED is the absorbed dose when given at infinitesimally small fraction doses or infinitesimally low dose rate. BED is greater or equal to D, so RE is greater than or equal to unity.

(172) Fig. 4.1 shows the value of RE for selected values of the different parameters in Eqs (4.14) and (4.13). For short effective half-lives, G approaches unity and RE

approaches a value valid for instantaneous delivery of the absorbed dose. For long effective half-times, G becomes small and RE approaches unity. Changes in D or α/β both result in variations of RE along the vertical axis, whereas changes in the repair half-life induce shifts along the horizontal direction.

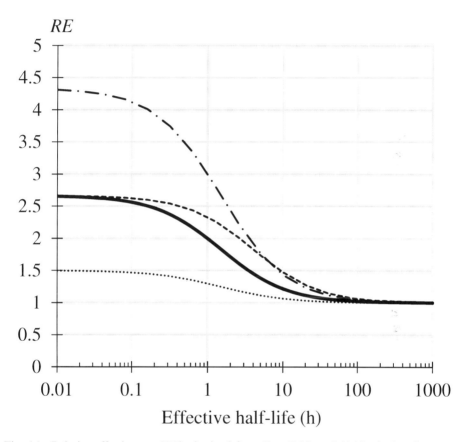

Fig. 4.1. Relative effectiveness (RE) obtained from Eqs (4.14) and (4.13). As baseline values, shown by the solid line, parameters used are $D = 5\,\mathrm{Gy}$, $\alpha/\beta = 3\,\mathrm{Gy}$, and $T_{\mathrm{rep}} = 1.5\,\mathrm{h}$. The dash-dotted line is obtained when the absorbed dose is changed to $10\,\mathrm{Gy}$, and the dotted line is obtained when α/β is changed to $10\,\mathrm{Gy}$. The dashed line is obtained when the repair half-time is changed to $4\,\mathrm{h}$.

5. SPECIFIC RADIOLOGICAL PROTECTION ISSUES

5.1. Introduction

(173) The use of radiation for radiopharmaceutical therapy is a planned exposure situation under regulatory control, with an appropriate authorisation in place from the regulatory body before the procedure may commence (ICRP, 2007a). Misadministration, spills, and other such incidents or accidents can give rise to potential exposure, but these remain part of the planned exposure situation as their occurrence is considered in the granting of an authorisation (Carlsson and LeHeron, 2014). Each of the categories of exposure of individuals (medical, occupational, and public) need to be considered in radiopharmaceutical therapy. In addition, the three fundamental principles of radiological protection (justification, optimisation, and limitation) (ICRP, 2007a) are applicable. In a nuclear medicine facility, occupational and public exposures are subject to all three principles, whereas medical exposure of patients is subject to the first two but not the third (ICRP, 2007b).

(174) Implementation of radiological protection for radiopharmaceutical therapy is an essential part of the system for implementing quality medical practice in a facility. The most important aspect is to establish a safety culture among staff, such that protection and accident prevention are regarded as important to daily activities. Several guidelines for implementation of radiological protection in a nuclear medicine facility have been developed (IAEA, 2005a,b, 2009, 2014a; Sisson et al., 2011) that address programme elements, responsibilities, education and training, facility design, monitoring, waste, and health surveillance.

5.2. Requirements for radiopharmaceutical therapy treatment rooms and wards

(175) The following aims should be considered in the design of radiopharmaceutical therapy treatment rooms and wards: optimising protection to reduce the exposure to external radiation and contamination, maintaining low radiation background levels to avoid interference with imaging equipment, meeting pharmaceutical requirements, sequestering waste appropriately, and ensuring safety and security of sources (locks and controlled access).

(176) Typically, rooms for high-activity patients should have separate toilet and washing facilities. Floors and other surfaces should be covered with smooth, continuous, non-absorbent, and non-porous surfaces that can be easily cleaned and decontaminated. The walls should be finished in a smooth and washable surface (e.g. painted with washable, non-porous paint). Secure areas should be provided with bins for the temporary storage of linen and waste contaminated with radioactivity.

(177) Proper shielding and ventilation is required for storage of bulk radioiodine containers. Preparation of activity for administration of radioiodine should be

performed in hoods with adequate air flow to protect staff, and extraction systems capable of adsorbing contaminants prior to emission. Adequate containment and exhaust should be provided for the storage of radioiodine waste and articles with residual contamination.

(178) Radiopharmaceutical therapy patients in unshielded hospital rooms may serve as radiation sources and expose people in adjacent areas to levels that might cause dose limits for the public to be exceeded. Vacating adjacent rooms or areas or installing shielding (such as permanent poured concrete, solid concrete block, steel plates, lead sheets, or portable shielding devices) may be necessary to ensure that public doses are maintained as low as reasonably achievable in adjacent areas (Chu et al., 2016). Areas on floors immediately above and below such patients' rooms, as well as on the same floor, must be considered. Table 5.1 gives typical shielding effectiveness values for ^{131}I which requires the most intensive shielding. Exposure or dose rates should be measured after each radiopharmaceutical administration to confirm that such exposures would not exceed a dose limit.

Table 5.1. Typical shielding effectiveness values for ^{131}I (CNSC, 2017).

	Half value layer[*]	Tenth value layer[†]
Lead	3.9 mm	12 mm
Steel	32 mm	64 mm
Concrete	118 mm	226 mm

[*]The thickness of shielding material required to reduce the unshielded dose rate to one-half of the original.
[†]The thickness of shielding material required to reduce the unshielded dose rate to one-tenth of the original.

(179) A monitoring system should be established in facilities, considering protection of the public and staff. For permanent shielding evaluations, it is important to design structural shielding properly, considering anticipated dose rates in controlled and supervised areas (IAEA, 2006b). Dose rates in occupied areas adjacent to the radionuclide treatment room should be monitored, and the results should be recorded to ensure that dose constraints are not exceeded and protection is optimised.

(180) Patient treatment rooms should ideally be for individual patients and adjacent to each other. Appropriate shielding may be required between adjacent treatment rooms (e.g. to reduce the exposure of workers) and between treatment rooms and other areas in order to minimise doses to members of the public as well as to staff. When required, additional shielding should be provided for nurses and visitors of radiopharmaceutical therapy patients; movable shields may be used within patient rooms. When required, prior to each treatment, movable shields should be placed close to the patient's bed in such a way that exposure of the nurses caring for the patient is minimised. Protection is achieved by anticipating the nurse's tasks, positions, and movements around the room.

5.3. Patients (medical exposure)

5.3.1. Justification and optimisation of protection

(181) In radiation therapy, the aim is to treat cancer or to palliate pain of the patient. The challenge of all radiation therapy is to optimise the relationship between the probability of tumour control and the risk of normal tissue complications. If the dose to the target tissue is too low, the therapy will be ineffective and the exposures will not have been sufficiently justified (ICRP, 2007b). However, the protection of organs and tissues outside the target volume is an integral part of treatment planning. Thus, the principle of optimisation of protection is applied to nuclear medicine therapeutic procedures that have been justified with an emphasis that the appropriate radiopharmaceutical and activity are selected, correctly calculated, measured, and administered so that the activity is primarily localised in the target of interest, while the activity in the rest of the body is maintained below levels that may be considered unacceptable in terms of adverse tissue reactions (ICRP, 2001b).

5.3.2. Considerations prior to therapy

(182) A risk assessment must be performed prior to radiopharmaceutical therapy to ensure that the patient is self-caring, able to tolerate isolation (if appropriate), and able to comply with radiation precautions (when necessary).

5.3.3. Pregnancy

(183) Pregnancy is a contraindication to radiopharmaceutical therapy, unless the therapy is life-saving. This advice is valid for radioiodine therapy and for other radionuclides with the potential to accumulate in fetal tissues. Beyond 10–13 weeks of gestation, the fetal thyroid may receive extremely high doses in cases of therapy using ^{131}I-iodide (Watson et al., 1989; Berg et al., 1998; ICRP, 2008). The possibility of pregnancy should be excluded before administration. Therefore, where treatment is likely or anticipated, the patient should also be advised to take appropriate contraceptive measures prior to therapy.

(184) Before any procedure using ionising radiation, it is important to determine whether a female patient is pregnant by performing a blood pregnancy test (Berg et al., 2008) before (usually within 72 h) treatment in all women, from menarche to 2 years after menopause, who could become pregnant. Surgical hysterectomy constitutes evidence that pregnancy is impossible and that a pregnancy test is not needed (Sisson et al., 2011).

(185) The feasibility and performance of medical exposures during pregnancy require specific consideration owing to the radiation sensitivity of the developing embryo/fetus (ICRP, 2001a, 2007a). ICRP has given detailed guidance in *Publications 84* (ICRP, 2000) and *105* (ICRP, 2007b). Radiation risks after prenatal radiation exposure are discussed in detail in *Publication 90* (ICRP, 2003).

(186) A problem occurs when a female who is not thought to be pregnant is treated for thyroid carcinoma, and is found to be pregnant after the administration of radioiodine. If a patient is discovered to be pregnant shortly after a therapeutic radioiodine administration, maternal hydration and frequent voiding should be encouraged to help eliminate maternal radioactivity and to reduce the residence time of radioiodine in the bladder. If the pregnancy is discovered within several hours of the radioiodine administration and the fetus is old enough to have a functional thyroid, one should consider thyroid blocking using potassium iodide. If the pregnancy is discovered later, the placental transfer of radioiodine can result in very high absorbed doses to the fetal thyroid that may cause significant damage. The fetal whole-body dose will usually be <100 mGy, and there is no reason to terminate the pregnancy on the grounds of potential adverse effects such as malformation or decreased intelligence (ICRP, 2000); however, the mother should be given replacement thyroid hormone, and consideration should be given to fetal thyroid effects, including risks of cancer.

5.3.4. Breast feeding

(187) Female patients should be advised that breast feeding is contraindicated after therapeutic administration of radionuclides. Any therapeutic radiopharmaceutical administered orally, intravenously, or arterially is potentially hazardous to the child, and breast feeding must cease. Intracavitary administrations of suspended particles such as ^{90}Y silicate represent little hazard of microspheres entering the mother's milk. Otherwise, breast feeding should be discontinued in patients receiving radiopharmaceutical therapy for two reasons: to prevent radionuclides in milk from reaching the infant (particularly the infant's thyroid gland in radioiodine therapies) (Azizi and Smyth, 2009); and to limit irradiation of the breast tissue, which may concentrate certain radionuclides during lactation. The restriction period depends on the radionuclide administered for therapy. In the case of ^{131}I treatment, the patient should stop breast feeding after the treatment until complete decay of the administered ^{131}I (Sisson et al., 2011).

5.3.5. Radioactive patients on dialysis

(188) The care of patients receiving radiopharmaceutical therapy who are on dialysis may require additional consideration, and radiological protection specialists or medical physicists should be consulted. For systemic treatments, these patients will not biologically clear radioactive materials in the same manner as typical patients as the clearance is highly dependent on the schedule of dialysis sessions.

5.3.6. Conception

(189) Conception should be avoided in both males and females, with clear advice from 4 to 12 months following radiopharmaceutical therapy. Table 5.2 obtained

from *Publication 106* (ICRP, 2004) gives additional information on precaution times for female avoidance of conception for specific radionuclide therapies. Pregnancy should also be delayed based on the need to normalise hormonal responses (in the case of thyroid therapy) for a successful pregnancy and healthy infant development, and to ensure that additional radiation treatment is not imminent (Sisson et al., 2011).

Table 5.2. Periods for avoiding pregnancy after radiopharmaceutical therapy to ensure that the dose to the fetus will not exceed 1 mGy.[*]

Radionuclide and form	Treatment of	All activities up to (MBq)	Avoid pregnancy (months)
^{131}I-iodide	Hyperthyroidism	800	4
^{131}I-iodide	Thyroid cancer	6000	4
^{131}I-mIBG	Neuroendocrine tumours	7500	3
^{32}P-phosphate	Myeloproliferative disease	200	3
^{89}Sr-chloride	Bone metastases	150	24
^{90}Y-colloid	Arthritic joints	400	0
^{90}Y-colloid	Malignancies	4000	1

[*]Selected data from Table 13.3 of *Publication 94* (ICRP, 2004).

(190) It is recommended, on the basis of general prudence, that male patients should avoid fathering children during the months immediately following therapy. However, no scientific evidence supports this view (Sawka et al., 2008a,b).

5.3.7. Prevention of medical errors with radiopharmaceuticals

(191) Accident prevention in radiation therapy should be an integral part of the design of equipment and premises, and of working procedures (ICRP, 2007b). A key feature of accident prevention has long been the use of multiple safeguards against the consequences of failures through design of equipment and facilities, as well as the use of working procedures. Working procedures should require key decisions, especially in radiation therapy, to be subject to independent confirmation. All services should develop and adopt criteria for checking of safety-critical steps in the referral, planning, optimisation, and delivery of therapy with radiopharmaceuticals. Effective communication between all staff and the patient is a vital part of the process. Remedial actions in emergency situations associated with the use of radioactive materials in therapy need to be identified prior to any programme launch (e.g. the dose from an excessive or erroneous administration of radioiodine in therapy may be reduced by the early administration of stable iodine as potassium iodide or iodate to reduce the uptake of radioiodine by the thyroid).

(192) Intravenous infusion of therapeutic radiopharmaceuticals must take place via an appropriate venous access device to ensure safe administration and prevent extravasation (Tennvall et al., 2007). Patients should be monitored for extravasation during infusion. In the event of extravasation, the infusion must be halted immediately. Extravasation can result in severe soft tissue lesions (van der Pol et al., 2017). Although there is no specific treatment, local hyperthermia, elevation of the extremity, and gentle massage may promote spreading of the radiopharmaceutical and reduce the local absorbed dose. The event must be recorded and follow-up is advised.

(193) Care should be exercised in avoiding administration of a therapeutic radiopharmaceutical to the wrong patient. In addition, prior to administration, the following should be verified to match the prescription:

- identification of the patient by two independent means;
- identity of the radionuclide;
- identity of the radiopharmaceutical;
- total activity;
- date and time of administration; and
- patients have been given information about their own safety.

(194) Records of the therapeutic radiopharmaceutical, data from dose planning, administered activity, date and time of administration, and verification of the initial and residual assay should be entered into the patient's medical record (ICRP, 2007b), together with the activity remaining in the patient at the time of discharge.

5.4. Staff (occupational exposure)

(195) Exposure of workers may arise from unsealed sources either through external irradiation of the body or through entry of radioactive substances into the body. The principles for the protection of workers from ionising radiation, including those in medicine, are discussed in *Publications 75* (ICRP, 1997) and *103* (ICRP, 2007a). Generally, the annual effective dose to staff working full-time in nuclear medicine with optimised protection should be <5 mSv. Facility and equipment design, proper shielding and handling of sources, and personal protective equipment and tools are important in protection (ICRP, 2008; Carlsson and LeHeron, 2014). Optimisation is also achieved through education and training (ICRP, 2009). Detailed requirements for protection against occupational exposure for nuclear medicine facilities are given in several publications (ICRP, 2007a,b; IAEA, 2011, 2014a), and recommendations on how to meet these requirements are given in IAEA Safety Guides (IAEA, 1999a,b,c) and, in particular, IAEA Safety Reports Series No. 40 (IAEA, 2005a).

(196) Pregnant women and individuals aged <18 years should not be involved in procedures with therapeutic levels of radiopharmaceuticals.

5.4.1. Protective equipment and tools

(197) Protective clothing should be used in radiopharmaceutical therapy areas where there is a likelihood of contamination. The clothing serves both to protect the body of the wearer and to help prevent the transfer of contamination to other areas. Protective clothing should be removed prior to going to other areas such as staff rooms. The protective clothing may include laboratory gowns, waterproof gloves, overshoes ('booties'), and caps and masks for aseptic work. Radiation safety glasses should be worn to protect the eyes from beta radiation and contamination of the eye. When beta emitters are handled, two layers of gloves should be worn to avoid contamination of the skin. There should be emphasis on the use of shielding, tools, and work practices that minimise exposure by preventing direct handling of vials, syringes, and contaminated articles.

(198) In radiopharmaceutical therapy, most occupational exposures come from ^{131}I, which emits 364-keV photons. The attenuation by a lead apron at this energy is minimal (less than a factor of 2), is unlikely to result in significant dose reduction, and may not justify the additional weight and discomfort of wearing such protective equipment. Wearing a lead apron to protect from ^{131}I could actually lead to an overall increase in exposure if individuals think that they are protected and stay near to sources or patients for longer periods. Thicker permanent or mobile lead shielding may be more effective in situations that warrant their use. Radiological protection experts and medical physicists should determine the need and types of shielding required for each situation. The use of automatic injection systems can reduce radiation dose to staff members (Rushforth et al., 2017).

(199) Administration is normally by the oral route, intravenous injection (systemic), intra-articular injection, or instillation of colloidal suspensions into closed body cavities (intracavitary). Shielded syringes should be utilised during the intravenous administration of radiopharmaceuticals to reduce extremity doses. Absorbent materials or pads should be placed underneath an injection or infusion site. The radiation protection officer at the facility should determine the need for these and other items of protective equipment (e.g. shoe covers, face shield) depending on circumstances.

(200) For oral administrations of therapeutic radiopharmaceuticals, the radioactive material should be placed in a shielded, spill-proof container. Care should be taken to minimise the chance for splashing liquid or for dropping capsules. Appropriate long-handled tools should be used when handling unshielded radioactive materials. For intravenous administrations by bolus injections, the syringe should be placed within a syringe shield (generally plastic for beta-emitting radionuclides to minimise bremsstrahlung, high Z materials for photon-emitting radionuclides) with a transparent window to allow for visualisation of the material in the syringe. For ^{90}Y radioimmunotherapy, a 5-mm-thick tungsten syringe shield has been shown to be slightly more protective than a 10-mm-thick plastic shield (Vanhavere et al., 2012). For intravenous administrations by slower drip or infusions, the activity container should be placed within a shield. For

high-energy photons, a significant thickness of lead or another high Z material may be needed.

(201) Procedures for administering a therapeutic radiopharmaceutical should include delivery of the prescribed therapeutic activity. Any residual activity in syringes, tubing, filters, or other equipment should be surveyed. Infusion pumps should be flushed or rinsed with isotonic saline (or other physiological buffer). All materials utilised in radionuclide administrations should be considered as medical and radioactive waste, and should be labelled with the radionuclide, a radiation precaution sticker, and stored and/or disposed of in a manner consistent with applicable regulations.

5.4.2. Individual monitoring

(202) Regular monitoring of external exposure should be performed during the management of patients receiving radiopharmaceutical therapy, and during preparation and administration of radiopharmaceuticals. Extremity monitoring should also be performed for people who handle radiopharmaceuticals (Rimpler et al., 2011; Sans-Merce et al., 2011).

(203) Significant doses to the hands can be received during preparation and administration of radiopharmaceuticals. If adequate protection measures are not in place, the exposure of the fingers will be high, particularly for high-energy beta radionuclides such as ^{90}Y (Barth and Mielcarek, 2002; Liepe et al., 2005a; Rimpler and Barth, 2007). The use of grasp forceps to hold the needle significantly reduces the dose to the hands (ICRP, 2008). Training and educational materials are provided by ICRP (http://www.icrp.org/page.asp?id=35) and other organisations (http://www.oramed-fp7.eu/en/Training%20material).

(204) Staff to be monitored in a nuclear medicine facility should include all those who work routinely with radionuclides, or nursing or other staff who spend time with therapy patients (ISO, 2016). Monitoring for internal contamination is rarely necessary in general nuclear medicine procedures unless a substantial intake is suspected (Carlsson and LeHeron, 2014). The circumstances in which internal monitoring become advisable are those where staff use significant quantities of ^{131}I for therapy. These staff should be included in a programme of regular thyroid uptake measurements.

5.4.3. Contamination control procedures

(205) In the event of a large-volume spill of radiopharmaceuticals, blood, urine, or vomitus, medical practitioners or staff should cover the spill with an absorbent material and contact the radiological protection experts/medical physicists immediately for appropriate clean-up assistance and specific instructions. After such a spillage, the following actions should be taken:

- the radiation protection officer should be informed immediately and should supervise the clean-up directly;

- absorbent pads should be placed over the spill to prevent further spread of contamination;
- all people not involved in the spill should leave the area immediately;
- access to the contaminated area should be restricted;
- all people involved in the spill should be monitored for contamination when leaving the room;
- if clothing is contaminated, it should be removed and placed in a plastic bag labelled 'radioactive';
- if contamination of skin occurs, the area should be washed immediately; and
- if contamination of an eye occurs, it should be flushed with large quantities of water.

(206) Upon discharge and release of the patient, all remaining waste and contaminated items should be removed and segregated into bags for disposable items and launderable items.

5.4.4. Surveys and monitoring

(207) For area monitoring, the operational quantity for assessing occupational effective dose is the ambient dose equivalent, $H^*(10)$ (ICRU, 1993; ICRP, 1996b, 2010). The ambient dose equivalent rate from the patient should be determined from personnel dosimeters. This information will assist in deriving appropriate arrangements for entry by visitors and staff, and for patient release. Rooms with radiotherapy patients should be controlled areas. In addition to dose rate monitoring, workplace contamination monitoring should be performed.

5.4.5. Emergency patient care

(208) Medical practitioners should provide all necessary medical care consistent with patient safety and appropriate medical management. Unless otherwise specified by the radiation protection officer at the facility, nurses, physicians, and other healthcare personnel should perform all routine duties, including those requiring direct patient contact, in a normal manner.

(209) Ward nurses should be informed when a patient may pose a radioactive hazard, and advice and training should be provided regularly.

(210) Radiological protection considerations should not prevent or delay lifesaving operations in the event that surgery is required. The following precautions should be observed:

- the operating room staff should be notified;
- operating procedures should be modified under the supervision of the radiation protection officer to minimise exposure and the spread of contamination;
- protective equipment may be used as long as efficiency and speed are not affected;

- rotation of personnel may be necessary if the surgical procedure is lengthy;
- the radiation protection officer should monitor all individuals involved; and
- doses to members of staff should be assessed, as may be required under the facility licence conditions.

(211) If the medical condition of a patient deteriorates such that intensive nursing care becomes necessary, such care is a priority and should not be delayed. However, the advice of the radiation protection officer should be sought immediately. In the event of deterioration in the patient's medical condition, frequent or continual monitoring of the patient may be necessary (e.g. septic shock, pulmonary oedema, stroke, or myocardial infarction).

(212) Life-saving efforts take precedence over consideration of radiation exposures received by medical personnel. This is particularly important for therapy patients containing large amounts of radionuclides. Medical personnel should, therefore, proceed with emergency care (e.g. when a patient has suffered a stroke), while taking precautions against the spread of contamination and minimising external exposure. The staff should avoid direct contact with the patient's mouth, and all members of the emergency team should wear protective gloves. Medical staff should be informed and trained on how to deal with radioactive patients. Rehearsals of the procedures should be held periodically.

5.4.6. Transfer of patients to another healthcare facility

(213) Some patients may need to be transferred to an alternate hospital, skilled nursing facility, nursing home, or hospice following radiopharmaceutical therapy. In such a case, care must be taken that, in addition to practical measures and advice to ensure the safety of other staff, compliance with any legal requirements relevant to the second institution is assured (IAEA, 2009). Patients transferred to another healthcare facility should meet the criteria for unrestricted clearance. However, the possibility for the generation of low-level radioactive waste should be examined by the radiation protection officer of the treating facility, and any issues should be discussed with the facility accepting the patient transfer. In the rare event that a patient being transferred to another healthcare facility does not meet the criteria for unrestricted clearance, the radiation protection officer should ensure that the facility accepting the patient transfer has an appropriate registration or licence that would allow acceptance of the patient with therapeutic amounts of radioactive materials on board. The radiation protection officer should provide radiation safety information and precautions, if any, for the patient and the receiving healthcare facility.

5.4.7. Death of a patient following radiopharmaceutical therapy

(214) In the event that a patient dies within the treating healthcare facility while still containing a therapeutic quantity of radioactive material, the treating medical practitioner and the radiation protection officer should be notified immediately.

Espenan et al. (1999) provided experience and guidance on radiological protection measures to be taken in the event of patient death.

(215) On the death of a radionuclide patient in a hospital, access to the room occupied by the deceased should be controlled until the room has been decontaminated and surveyed. Identification of the possibility that a body may contain radioactive substances relies on information provided in the patient records, the information card, or information gleaned from relatives or others. A body bag may need to be used to contain leakage of radioactive substances. To minimise external radiation, the body may need to be retained in a controlled area.

(216) Applicable dose limits apply to members of the public and radiation workers that must care for the deceased patient.

(217) Unsealed radioactive substances may be present in a particular body cavity or organ, or they may have concentrated after systemic administration (such as residual ^{131}I in the thyroid). Drainage of the cavity or excision of the organ may reduce exposure if undertaken at the start of the autopsy. In addition, care should be taken with respect to organs with significant activity. In cases where the patient had received a dose of beta-emitting colloid or spheres (e.g. ^{32}P-phosphate into a body cavity or ^{90}Y microspheres into the liver), significant activity may be present in the cavity fluid or the embolised organ. Beta-radiation sources may provide significant dose to the hands because they will be in close contact with body tissues and fluids (NCRP, 2006). Autopsy and pathology staff should wear standard protective clothing (e.g. gloves, laboratory coat, and eye protection) and personnel monitoring should be considered. For beta emitters, double surgical gloves may be helpful in reducing skin contact. Face shields may be employed to prevent liquids from splashing on to the face.

(218) A portion of the activity retained will appear in cremated remains, and may be sufficient, particularly in the case of long-lived radionuclides, to require controls to be specified. The main concern is in respect to the scattering of ashes, although contact dose rates with the container may have to be considered if cremation takes place shortly after administration.

(219) Crematorium employees may receive external exposure from the radioactive body or from contamination of the crematorium, or internal exposure from inhalation of radioactive particles while handling the ashes (Wallace and Bush, 1991). Bodies that contain gamma-emitting radionuclides may result in slight external exposure to crematorium employees.

(220) The most likely potential concern for the general population in the vicinity of the crematorium is inhalation of radioactive material emitted with the stack gases.

5.5. Comforters and carers (medical exposure), and members of the public (public exposure)

(221) *Publication 94* (ICRP, 2004) recommends that young children and infants, as well as visitors not engaged in direct care or comforting, should be treated as members of the public and should be subject to the public dose limit of 1 mSv year^{-1}. The

registrant or licensee is responsible for controlling public exposure resulting from a nuclear medicine practice (IAEA, 2011).

(222) While medical exposures are predominantly delivered to individuals (patients), other individuals caring for and comforting patients are also exposed to radiation. These individuals include parents and others, normally family or close friends, who may come close to patients following administration of radiopharmaceuticals. These exposures are considered as medical exposures (ICRP, 2007a). *Publication 94* (ICRP, 2004) recommends that for individuals directly involved in comforting and caring (other than young children and infants), a dose constraint of 5 mSv per episode (for the duration of a given release from hospital after therapy) is reasonable.

5.5.1. Release of the patient

(223) A patient who has undergone a therapeutic nuclear medicine procedure represents a potential source of radiation to others in close proximity to the patient. Excreta and vomitus result in the possibility of contamination of the patient's environments.

(224) If individuals are not occupationally exposed and they knowingly and willingly provide care to the patient, they should be classified as a comforter and carer. Their exposure is considered part of medical exposure, and they are not subject to dose limits but to dose constraints (ICRP, 2007b). If the person is simply a member of the public, including people whose work in the nuclear medicine facility does not involve working with radiation, their exposure is part of public exposure.

(225) Patients do not need to be hospitalised automatically after all radionuclide therapies. Relevant national dose limits must be met and the principle of optimisation of protection must be applied, including the use of relevant dose constraints. The decision to hospitalise or to release a patient should be determined on an individual basis considering factors such as the radiation level of the patient measured by dose rate monitoring, the residual activity in the patient, the patient's wishes, family considerations (particularly the presence of children), environmental factors, and existing guidance and regulations. Hospitalisation will reduce exposure to the public and relatives, but will increase overall cost and may increase exposure to hospital staff. Hospitalisation often involves a significant psychological burden, as well as monetary and other costs that should be analysed and justified. *Publication 94* gives detailed recommendations related to release of patients after therapy with unsealed radionuclides (ICRP, 2004).

(226) Current recommendations regarding release of patients after therapy with unsealed radionuclides vary widely around the world. However, the decision to release a patient is based on the assumption that the risk can be controlled when the patients return to their homes. This is generally achieved by combining an appropriate release criterion with well-tailored instructions and information for the patients that will allow them to deal effectively with the potential risks.

(227) When appropriate, the patient or legal guardian must be provided with written and verbal instructions with a view to the restriction of doses to people in contact with the patient as far as reasonably achievable, and information on the risks of ionising radiation. Specific instructions should include minimisation of the spread of contamination, minimisation of exposure to family members, cessation of breast feeding, and delaying conception after therapy. Procedures for advising carers and comforters should be in place, developed in consultation with the radiation protection officer. Registrants and licensees should ensure that carers and comforters of patients during the course of treatment with radionuclides receive sufficient written instructions on relevant radiological protection precautions (e.g. time and proximity to the patient). Example methodologies for evaluating precaution time requirements have been published (Zanzonico et al., 2000; NCRP, 2006; IAEA, 2009; Sisson et al., 2011).

5.5.2. Visitors to patients

(228) Visitors are not normally admitted into the patient's hospital room after a high-dose radionuclide therapy. Licensees should also take measures to restrict public exposure to contamination in areas accessible to the public.

5.5.3. Travel

(229) Travel following therapy should be within certain restrictions, and patients should carry relevant documentation in case of a medical emergency. If travelling, it should be noted that radiation detectors used for security purposes (e.g. in airports) are sufficiently sensitive to detect low levels of radiation.

(230) If the patient must ride or drive with another person, time and distance constraints apply. Use of a larger vehicle, such as a van, would permit further separation and consequently a reduction in exposure to others. ICRP has previously evaluated the potential doses to others during patient travel, and has published recommendations that allow the use of public transportation by some patients treated with nuclear medicine therapy (ICRP, 2004, Table 10.7). Radionuclide characteristics and activity administered should be considered. For example, for patients treated for hyperthyroidism, the patient may use public transportation for up to 0.5 h if treated with 800 MBq or up to 3.5 h if treated with 200 MBq (ICRP, 2004).

(231) Patients travelling after radioiodine therapy rarely present a hazard to other passengers if travel times are limited to a few hours. Travel for 1–2 h immediately after treatment is permissible in a private automobile large enough for the patient to maintain a distance ≥ 1 m from other occupants. A case-by-case analysis is necessary to determine the actual travel restrictions for each patient, especially for longer trips and for travel by public transport. A stay in a hotel or motel is not recommended after treatment with nuclear medicine therapy without assessment of the potential ramification on radiation exposure to members of the public.

(232) International security measures, such as at airports and border crossing points, may include extremely sensitive radiation detectors. Released patients with residual activity may trigger the alarms. With current technology, it is possible to detect ^{131}I activity as low as 0.01 MBq at 2–3 m (Dauer et al., 2007a). It is possible that patients treated with radionuclides could trigger alarms for $\geq$95 days (Dauer et al., 2007b,c). Triggering of an alarm does not mean that a patient is emitting dangerous levels of radiation, as the detectors are designed to detect levels of radio-activity far below those of concern to human health. The security authorities understand that released patients may alarm at check points. Personnel operating such detectors should be specifically trained to identify and deal with nuclear medicine patients. Records of the specific details of therapy with unsealed radionuclides should be maintained at the hospital and given to the patient, along with written precautionary instructions (ICRP, 2008).

(233) If travel is planned within 4 months of receiving radiopharmaceutical therapy, particularly across international borders or via airports, tunnels, or over bridges or whenever inspection is likely, a form or card should be provided to the patient (Sisson et al., 2011). The form should specify the date of treatment, the radionuclide activity administered, the treating facility, and the name and telephone number of a contact individual knowledgeable about the case.

5.5.4. Radioactive waste

(234) Licensees are responsible for ensuring that the optimisation of radiological protection takes into account the discharge of radioactive substances from a source to the environment (IAEA, 2000, 2004, 2005a). Radioactive waste for short-lived medical isotopes should be contained in appropriate storage areas through complete decay. Much of the administered activity is eventually discharged to public sewer systems. Storage of a patient's excreta is not necessary (ICRP, 2004); however, local restrictions regarding the discharge of activity may apply. Once a patient has been released from hospital, the excreted radioactivity levels are low enough to be discharged through the home toilet without approaching public dose limits.

6. SUMMARY OF RECOMMENDATIONS

(235) The increasing use of radiopharmaceuticals for cancer therapy promises new treatment options for patients. The challenge for all radiation therapy is to optimise the ability to treat cancer successfully (tumour control probability) against potential adverse effects and normal tissue complications. Radiopharmaceutical therapy provides opportunities to maximise the therapeutic index, a measure of both efficacy and safety.

(236) In radiopharmaceutical therapy, the absorbed dose to an organ or tissue is governed by the individual patient biokinetics (uptake, retention, and clearance), which may vary widely from one patient to another. Measurements of radiopharmaceutical biokinetics provide essential information needed for internal dose assessment.

(237) Due to biokinetic differences, personalised dosimetry must be performed for each patient. In principle, a fully personalised approach based on patient-specific measurements can ensure treatment with an appropriate activity level without exceeding normal organ and tissue toxicity thresholds.

(238) Special consideration should be given to pregnant women. Pregnancy is contraindicated in radiopharmaceutical therapy, unless the therapy is life-saving. Female patients should be advised that breast feeding is also contraindicated after therapeutic administration of radionuclides.

(239) In addition to the patients treated with radiopharmaceutical therapy, the people at risk of exposure include hospital staff, members of the patient's family (including children), carers, neighbours, and the general public. These risks can be effectively managed and mitigated with well-trained staff, appropriate facilities, and the use of patient-specific radiation safety precaution instructions.

(240) Radiological protection measures to minimise medical staff exposures include use of proper equipment and shielding, safe handling of radioactive sources, use of personal protective equipment and tools, and education and training for commitment to improve awareness and engagement in safety practice. Individual monitoring of the worker doses and extremity doses must be considered during the management of radiopharmaceutical therapy patients, and during preparation and administration of the radiopharmaceuticals.

(241) Medical practitioners should provide all necessary medical care consistent with patient safety and appropriate medical management. Radiological protection considerations should not prevent or delay life-saving operations in the event that surgery is required. Staff should be informed when a patient may present a source of radiation exposure. Training should help the staff to put risk concerns into proper perspective.

(242) The decision to hospitalise or release a patient after therapy should be made on an individual basis, considering factors such as the residual activity in the patient and existing guidance and regulations. Specific radiological protection precautions should be provided to patients and carers.

(243) Prevention of medical errors with radiopharmaceuticals should be an integral part of the design of equipment and premises, and of the working procedures.

REFERENCES

Alexander, E.K., Pearce, E.N., Brent, G.A., et al., 2017. 2017 Guidelines of the American Thyroid Association for the diagnosis and management of thyroid disease during pregnancy and the postpartum. Thyroid 27, 315–389.

Andersson, H., Cederkrantz, E., Bäck, T., et al., 2009. Intraperitoneal alpha-particle radioimmunotherapy of ovarian cancer patients: pharmacokinetics and dosimetry of ^{211}At-MX35 F(ab')2 – a phase I study. J. Nucl. Med. 50, 1153–1160.

Andersson, M., Johansson, L., Minarik, D., et al., 2014. An internal radiation dosimetry computer program, IDAC 2.0, for estimation of patient doses from radiopharmaceuticals. Radiat. Prot. Dosim. 162, 299–305.

Ansell, B.M., Crook, A., Mallard, J.R., et al., 1963. Evaluation of intra-articular colloidal gold Au 198 in the treatment of persistent knee effusions. Ann. Rheum. Dis. 22, 435–439.

Azizi, F., Smyth, P., 2009. Breastfeeding and maternal and infant iodine nutrition. Clin. Endocrinol. 70, 803–809.

Barbet, J., Bardies, M., Bourgeois, M., et al., 2012. Radiolabeled antibodies for cancer imaging and therapy. Methods Mol. Biol. 907, 681–697.

Barendsen, G.W., 1982. Dose fractionation, dose rate and iso-effect relationships for normal tissue responses. Int. J. Radiat. Oncol. Biol. Phys. 8, 1981–1997.

Barone, R., Borson-Chazot, F.O., Valkerna, R., et al., 2005. Patient-specific dosimetry in predicting renal toxicity with Y-90-DOTATOC: relevance of kidney volume and dose rate in finding a dose–effect relationship. J. Nucl. Med. 46 (Suppl. 1), 99S–106S.

Barth, I., Mielcarek, J., 2002. Occupational Beta Radiation Exposure During Radiosynoviorthesis. Sixth European ALARA Network Workshop in Occupational Exposure Optimization in Medical Field and Radiopharmaceutical Industry, 23–25 October 2002, Madrid, Spain, pp. 43–46. Available at: http://www.eu-alara.net/images/stories/pdf/program6/Session%20B/I_Barth.pdf (last accessed 8 April 2019).

Benua, R.S., Cicale, N.R., Sonenberg, M., et al., 1962. The relation of radioiodine dosimetry to results and complications in the treatment of metastatic thyroid cancer. Am. J. Roentgenol. Radium Ther. Nucl. Med. 87, 171–182.

Bentzen, S.M., Dorr, W., Gahbauer, R., et al., 2012. Bioeffect modeling and equieffective dose concepts in radiation oncology – terminology, quantities and units. Radiother. Oncol. 105, 266–268.

Berg, G., Nystrom, E., Jacobsson, L., et al., 1998. Radioiodine treatment of hyperthyroidism in a pregnant woman. J. Nucl. Med. 39, 357–361.

Berg, G., Jacobsson, L., Nyström, E., et al., 2008. Consequences of inadvertent radioiodine treatment of Graves' disease and thyroid cancer in undiagnosed pregnancy. Can we rely on routine pregnancy testing? Acta Oncol. 47, 145–149.

Bodei, L., Cremonesi, M., Ferrari, M., et al., 2008. Long-term evaluation of renal toxicity after peptide receptor radionuclide therapy with Y-90-DOTATOC and Lu-177-DOTATATE: the role of associated risk factors. Eur. J. Nucl. Med. Mol. Imaging 35, 1847–1856.

Bodei, L., Mueller-Brand, J., Baum, R.P., et al., 2013. The joint IAEA, EANM, and SNMMI practical guidance on peptide receptor radionuclide therapy (PRRNT) in neuroendocrine tumours. Eur. J. Nucl. Med. Mol. Imaging 40, 800–816.

Bolch, W.E., Eckerman, K.F., Sgouros, G., et al., 2009. MIRD Pamphlet No. 21: a generalized schema for radiopharmaceutical dosimetry – standardization of nomenclature. J. Nucl. Med. 50, 477–484.

Bowring, C.S., Keeling, D.H., 1978. Absorbed radiation dose in radiation synovectomy. Br. J. Radiol. 51, 836–837.

Brandt, L., Anderson, H., 1995. Survival and risk of leukaemia in polycythemia vera and essential thrombocythemia treated with oral radiophosphorus. Eur. J. Haematol. 54, 21–26.

Breen, S.L., Powe, J.E., Porter, A.T., 1992. Dose estimation in strontium-89 radiotherapy of metastatic prostatic carcinoma. J. Nucl. Med. 33, 1316–1323.

Brown, A.P., Chen, J., Hitchcock, Y.J., et al., 2008. The risk of second primary malignancies up to three decades after the treatment of differentiated thyroid cancer. J. Clin. Endocrinol. Metabol. 93, 504–515.

Buckley, S.E., Chittenden, S.J., Saran, F.H., et al., 2009. Whole-body dosimetry for individualized treatment planning of ^{131}I-MIBG radionuclide therapy for neuroblastoma. J. Nucl. Med. 50, 1518–1524.

Bushnell, D.L. Jr, O'Dorisio, T.M., O'Dorisio, M.S., et al., 2010. ^{90}Y-edotreotide for metastatic carcinoid refractory to octreotide. J. Clin. Oncol. 28, 1652–1659.

Carlier, T., Willowson, K.P., Fourkal, E., et al., 2015. ^{90}Y-PET imaging: exploring limitations and accuracy under conditions of low counts and high random fraction. Med. Phys. 42, 4295–4309.

Carlsson, S., LeHeron, J., 2014. Radiation protection. In: Bailey, D., Humm, J., Todd-Pokropek, A., et al. (Eds.), Nuclear Medicine Physics: a Handbook for Teachers and Students. International Atomic Energy Agency, Vienna.

Chatal, J.F., Faivre-Chauvet, A., Bardies, M., et al., 1995. Bifunctional antibodies for radioimmunotherapy. Hybridoma 14, 125–128.

Chatal, J.F., Kraeber-Bodere, F., Barbet, J., 2008. Consolidation radioimmunotherapy of follicular lymphoma: a step towards cure? Eur. J. Nucl. Med. Mol. Imaging 35, 1236–1239.

Chiesa, C., Maccauro, M., Romito, R., et al., 2011. Need, feasibility and convenience of dosimetric treatment planning in liver selective internal radiation therapy with Y-90 microspheres: the experience of the National Cancer Institute of Milan. Q. J. Nucl. Med. Mol. Imaging 55, 168–197.

Chittendsen, S.J., Hindorf, C., Parker, C.C., et al., 2015. A phase 1, open-label study of the biodistribution, pharmacokinetics, and dosimetry of 223Ra-dichloride in patients with hormone-refractory prostate cancer and skeletal metastases. J. Nucl. Med. 56, 1304–1309.

Chu, B.P., Horan, C., Basu, E., et al., 2016. Feasibility of administering high-dose ^{131}I-MIBG therapy to children with high-risk neurobastoma without lead-lined rooms. Pediatr. Blood Cancer. 63, 801–807.

CNSC, 2017. Radionuclide Information Booklet. Canadian Nuclear Safety Commission, Ottawa. Available at: https://nuclearsafety.gc.ca/pubs_catalogue/uploads/Radionuclide-Information-Booklet-2016-eng.pdf (last accessed 8 April 2018).

Cremonesi, M., Ferrari, M., Bodei, L., et al., 2006a. Dosimetry in peptide radionuclide receptor therapy: a review. J. Nucl. Med. 47, 1467–1475.

Cremonesi, M., Ferrari, M., Paganelli, G., et al., 2006b. Radiation protection in radionuclide therapies with ^{90}Y-conjugates: risk and safety. Eur. J. Nucl. Med. Mol. Imaging 33, 1321–1327.

Cremonesi, M., Ferrari, M., Grana, C.M., et al., 2007. High-dose radioimmunotherapy with ^{90}Y-ibritumomab tiuxetan: comparative dosimetric study for tailored treatment. J. Nucl. Med. 48, 1871–1879.

Cremonesi, M., Botta, F., Di Dia, A., et al., 2010. Dosimetry for treatment with radiolabelled somatostatin analogues. A review. Q. J. Nucl. Med. Mol. Imaging 54, 37–51.

Cremonesi, M., Chiesa, C., Strigari, L., et al., 2014. Radioembolization of hepatic lesions from a radiobiology and dosimetric perspective. Front. Oncol. 4, 210.

Dale, R.G., 1996. Dose-rate effects in targeted radiotherapy. Phys. Med. Biol. 41, 1871–1884.

D'Angelo, G., Sciuto, R., Salvatori, M., et al., 2012. Targeted "bone-seeking" radiopharmaceuticals for palliative treatment of bone metastases: a systematic review and meta-analysis. Q. J. Nucl. Med. Mol. Imaging 56, 538–543.

Das, B., 2007. Role of radiosynovectomy in the treatment of rheumatoid arthritis and hemophilic arthropathies. Biomed. Imaging Interv. J. 3, e45.

Dauer, L.T., St. Germain, J., Williamson, M.J., et al., 2007a. Whole-body clearance kinetics and external dosimetry of [131]I-3F8 monoclonal antibody for radioimmunotherapy of neuroblastoma. Health Phys. 92, 33–39.

Dauer, L.T., Williamson, M.J., St. Germain, J., et al., 2007b. Tl-201 stress tests and homeland security. J. Nucl. Cardiol. 14, 582–588.

Dauer, L.T., Strauss, H.W., St. Germain, J., 2007c. Responding to nuclear granny. J. Nucl. Cardiol. 14, 904–905.

Dauer, L.T., Williamson, M.J., Humm, J., et al., 2014. Radiation safety considerations for the use of [223]RaCl$_2$ in men with castration-resistant prostate cancer. Health Phys. 106, 494–504.

Delpon, G., Ferrer, L., Lisbona, A., et al., 2002. Correction of count losses due to deadtime on a DST-XLi (SMVi-GE) camera during dosimetric studies in patients injected with iodine-131. Phys. Med. Biol. 47, N79–N90.

Dewaraja, Y.K., Frey, E.C., Sgouros, G., et al., 2012. MIRD Pamphlet No. 23: quantitative SPECT for patient-specific 3-dimensional dosimetry in internal radionuclide therapy. J. Nucl. Med. 53, 1310–1325.

Dewaraja, Y.K., Ljungberg, M., Green, A.J., et al., 2013. MIRD Pamphlet No. 24: guidelines for quantitative ^{131}I SPECT in dosimetry applications. J. Nucl. Med. 54, 2182–2188.

Eary, J.F., Collins, C., Stabin, M., et al., 1993. Samarium-153-EDTMP biodistribution and dosimetry estimation. J. Nucl. Med. 34, 1031–1036.

Espenan, G.D., Nelson, J.A., Fisher, D.R., et al., 1999. Experiences with high dose radiopeptide therapy: the health physics perspective. Health Phys. 76, 225–235.

Fernández Tomás, M., Preylowski, V., Schlögl, S., et al., 2012. Influence of the reconstruction parameters on image quantification with SPECT/CT. Eur. J. Nucl. Med. Mol. Imaging 39, S254.

Finlay, I.G., Mason, M.D., Shelley, M., 2005. Radioisotopes for the palliation of metastatic bone cancer: a systematic review. Lancet Oncol. 6, 392–400.

Fisher, D.R., Meredith, R.F., Shen, S., 2009. MIRD dose estimate report No. 20: radiation absorbed dose estimates for [111]In- and ^{90}Y-ibritumomab tiuxetan (Zevalin[TM]). J. Nucl. Med. 44, 465–474.

Flower, M.A., Al-Saadi, A., Harmer, C.L., et al., 1994. Dose–response study on thyrotoxic patients undergoing positron emission tomography and radioiodine therapy. Eur. J. Nucl. Med. Mol. Imaging 21, 531–536.

Flux, G.D., Haq, M., Chittenden, S.J., et al., 2010. A dose–effect correlation for radioiodine ablation in differentiated thyroid cancer. Eur. J. Nucl. Med. Mol. Imaging 37, 270–275.

Flux, G.D., Chittenden, S.J., Saran, F., et al., 2011. Clinical applications of dosimetry for mIBG therapy. Q. J. Nucl. Med. Mol. Imaging 55, 116–125.

Fowler, J.F., 1989. The linear-quadratic formula and progress in fractionated radiotherapy. Br. J. Radiol. 62, 679–694.

Francis, G.L., Waguespack, S.G., Bauer, A.J., et al., 2015. Management guidelines for children with thyroid nodules and differentiated thyroid cancer. Thyroid. 25, 716–759.

Franzius, C., Dietlein, M., Biermann, M., et al., 2007. [Procedure guideline for radioiodine therapy and [131]iodine whole-body scintigraphy in paediatric patients with differentiated thyroid cancer]. Nuklearmedizin 46, 224–231.

Gains, J.E., Bomanji, J.B., Fersht, N.L., et al., 2011. ^{177}Lu-DOTATATE molecular radiotherapy for childhood neuroblastoma. J. Nucl. Med. 52, 1041–1047.

Garaventa, A., Bellagamba, O., Lo Piccolo, M.S., et al., 1999. I-131-metaiodobenzylguanidine (I-131-MIBG) therapy for residual neuroblastoma: a mono-institutional experience with 43 patients. Br. J. Cancer 81, 1378–1384.

Gaze, M.N., Chang, Y.C., Flux, G.D., et al., 2005. Feasibility of dosimetry-based high-dose ^{131}I-meta-iodobenzylguanidine with topotecan as a radiosensitizer in children with metastatic neuroblastoma. Cancer Biother. Radiopharm. 20, 195–199.

Gear, J.I., Cox, M.G., Gustafsson, J., et al., 2018. EANM practical guidance on uncertainty analysis for molecular radiotherapy absorbed dose calculations. Eur. J. Nucl. Med. Mol. Imaging 45, 2456–2474.

George, S.L., Falzone, N., Chittenden, S., et al., 2016. Individualized ^{131}I-mIBG therapy in the management of refractory and relapsed neuroblastoma. Nucl. Med. Commun. 37, 466–472.

Giammarile, F., Chiti, A., Lassmann, M., et al., 2008. EANM procedure guideline for ^{131}I-meta-iodobenzylguanidine (^{131}I-mIBG) therapy. Eur. J. Nucl. Med. Mol. Imaging 35, 1039–1047.

Giammarile, F., Bodei, L., Chiesa, C., et al., 2011. EANM procedure guideline for the treatment of liver cancer and liver metastases with intra-arterial radioactive compounds. Eur. J. Nucl. Med. Mol. Imaging 38, 1393–1406.

Glatting, G., Landmann, M., Kull, T., et al., 2005. Internal radionuclide therapy: the ULMDOS software for treatment planning. Med. Phys. 32, 2399–2405.

Glatting, G., Lassmann, M., 2007. Nuklearmedizinische dosimetrie. In: Krause, B-J., Schwaiger, M., Buck, A.K. (Eds.), Nuklearmedizinische Onkologie. Hüthig Jehle Rehm, Landsberg.

Gleisner, K.S., Brolin, G., Sundlov, A., et al., 2015. Long-term retention of ^{177}Lu/[177m]Lu-dotatate in patients investigated by gamma-spectrometry and gamma-camera imaging. J. Nucl. Med. 56, 976–984.

Goldenberg, D.M., Chang, C.H., Rossi, E.A., et al., 2012. Pretargeted molecular imaging and radioimmunotherapy. Theranostics 2, 523–540.

Goldsmith, S.J., 2010. Radioimmunotherapy of lymphoma: Bexxar and Zevalin. Semin. Nucl. Med. 40, 122–135.

Grassi, E., Sghedoni, R., Asti, M., et al., 2009. Radiation protection in ^{90}Y-labelled DOTA-D-Phe1-Tyr$_3$-octreotide preparations. Nucl. Med. Commun. 30, 176–182.

Gustafsson, J., Nilsson, P., Gleisner, K.S., 2013a. On the biologically effective dose (BED) – using convolution for calculating the effects of repair: I. Analytical considerations. Phys. Med. Biol. 58, 1507–1527.

Gustafsson, J., Nilsson, P., Gleisner, K.S., 2013b. On the biologically effective dose (BED) – using convolution for calculating the effects of repair: II. Numerical considerations. Phys. Med. Biol. 58, 1529–1548.

Guy, M.J., Flux, G.D., Papavasileiou, P., et al., 2003. A dedicated package for ^{131}I SPECT quantification, registration and patient-specific dosimetry. Cancer Biother. Radiopharm. 18, 61–69.

Hanaoka, K., Hosono, M., Tatsumi, Y., et al., 2015. Heterogeneity of intratumoral ^{111}In-ibritumomab tiuxetan and ^{18}F-FDG distribution in association with therapeutic response in radioimmunotherapy for B-cell non-Hodgkin's lymphoma. EJNMI Res. 5, 10.

Hänscheid, H., Lassmann, M., Luster, M., et al., 2006. Iodine biokinetics and dosimetry in radioiodine therapy of thyroid cancer: procedures and results of a prospective international controlled study of ablation after rhTSH or hormone withdrawal. J. Nucl. Med. 47, 648–654.

Hänscheid, H., Lassmann, M., Luster, M., et al., 2009. Blood dosimetry from a single measurement of the whole body radioiodine retention in patients with differentiated thyroid carcinoma. Endocr. Relat. Cancer 16, 1283–1289.

Hänscheid, H., Canzi, C., Eschner, W., et al., 2013. EANM Dosimetry Committee series on standard operational procedures for pre-therapeutic dosimetry. II. Dosimetry prior to radioiodine therapy of benign thyroid diseases. Eur. J. Nucl. Med. Mol. Imaging 40, 1126–1134.

Haugen, B.R., Alexander, E.K., Bible, K.C., et al., 2016. 2015 American Thyroid Association management guidelines for adult patients with thyroid nodules and differentiated thyroid cancer: the American Thyroid Association Guidelines Task Force on Thyroid Nodules and Differentiated Thyroid Cancer. Thyroid 26, 1–133.

Hay, I.D., Gonzalez-Losada, T., Reinalda, M.S., et al., 2010. Long-term outcome in 215 children and adolescents with papillary thyroid cancer treated during 1940 through 2008. World J. Surg. 34, 1192–1202.

Hindorf, C., Chittenden, S., Causer, L., et al., 2007. Dosimetry for ^{90}Y-DOTATOC therapies in patients with neuroendocrine tumors. Cancer Biother. Radiopharmaceut. 22, 130–135.

Hindorf, C., Glatting, G., Chiesa, C., et al., 2010. EANM Dosimetry Committee guidelines for bone marrow and whole-body dosimetry. Eur. J. Nucl. Med. Mol. Imaging 37, 1238–1250.

Hoefnagel, C.A., Voute, P.A., De Kraker, J., et al., 1991. [^{131}I]metaiodobenzylguanidine therapy after conventional therapy for neuroblastoma. J. Nucl. Biol. Med. 35, 202–206.

Honarvar, H., Westerlund, K., Altai, A., et al., 2016. Feasibility of affibody molecule-based PNA-mediated radionuclide pretargeting of malignant tumors. Theranostics 6, 93–103.

Howarth, D., Epstein, M., Lan, L., et al., 2001. Determination of the optimal minimum radioiodine dose in patients with Graves' disease: a clinical outcome study. Eur. J. Nucl. Med. 28, 1489–1495.

Howell, R.W., Goddu, S.M., Dandamundi, V.R., 1994. Application of the linear-quadratic model to radioimmunotherapy: further support for the advantage of longer-lived radionuclides. J. Nucl. Med. 35, 1861–1869.

IAEA, 1999a. Occupational Protection. IAEA Safety Standards Series No. RS-G-1.1. International Atomic Energy Agency, Vienna.

IAEA, 1999b. Assessment of Occupational Exposure Due to Intakes of Radionuclides. IAEA Safety Standards Series No. RS-G-1.2. International Atomic Energy Agency, Vienna.

IAEA, 1999c. Assessment of Occupational Exposure Due to External Sources of Radiation. IAEA Safety Standards Series No. RS-G-1.3. International Atomic Energy Agency, Vienna.

IAEA, 2000. Regulatory Control of Radioactive Discharges to the Environment. IAEA Safety Standards Series No. WS-G-2.3. International Atomic Energy Agency, Vienna.

IAEA, 2004. Applications of the Concepts of Exclusion, Exemption and Clearance. IAEA Safety Standards Series No. RS-G-1.7. International Atomic Energy Agency, Vienna.

IAEA, 2005a. Applying Radiation Safety Standards in Nuclear Medicine. Safety Reports Series No. 40. International Atomic Energy Agency, Vienna.

IAEA, 2005b. Management of Waste from the Use of Radioactive Material in Medicine, Industry, Agriculture, Research and Education. IAEA Safety Standards Series No. WS-G-2.7. International Atomic Energy Agency, Vienna.

IAEA, 2006a. Application of the Management System for Facilities and Activities: Safety Guide. IAEA Safety Standards Series No. GS-G-3.1. International Atomic Energy Agency, Vienna.

IAEA, 2006b. Radiation Protection in the Design of Radiotherapy Facilities. Safety Report Series No. 47. International Atomic Energy Agency, Vienna.

IAEA, 2009. Release of Patients After Radionuclide Therapy. Safety Reports Series No. 63. International Atomic Energy Agency, Vienna.

IAEA, 2011. Radiation Protection and Safety of Radiation Sources: International Basic Safety Standards – Interim Edition. IAEA Safety Standards Series No. GSR Part 3 (Interim). International Atomic Energy Agency, Vienna.

IAEA, 2014a. Nuclear Medicine Physics: a Handbook for Teachers and Students. International Atomic Energy Agency, Vienna.

IAEA, 2014b. Quantitative Nuclear Medicine Imaging: Concepts, Requirements and Methods. IAEA Human Health Reports No. 9. International Atomic Energy Agency, Vienna.

ICRP, 1987. Radiation dose to patients from radiopharmaceuticals. ICRP Publication 53. Ann. ICRP 18(1–4).

ICRP, 1996a. Radiological protection and safety in medicine. ICRP Publication 73. Ann. ICRP 26(2).

ICRP, 1996b. Conversion coefficients for use in radiological protection against external radiation. ICRP Publication 74. Ann. ICRP 26(3/4).

ICRP, 1997. General principles for the radiation protection of workers. ICRP Publication 75. Ann. ICRP 27(1).

ICRP, 1998. Radiation dose to patients from radiopharmaceuticals (Addendum 2 to ICRP Publication 53). ICRP Publication 80. Ann. ICRP 28(3).

ICRP, 2000. Pregnancy and medical radiation. ICRP Publication 84. Ann. ICRP 30(1).

ICRP, 2001a. Doses to the embryo and fetus from intakes of radionuclide by the mother. ICRP Publication 88. Ann. ICRP 31(1–3).

ICRP, 2001b. Radiation and your patient – a guide for medical practitioners. ICRP Supporting Guidance 2. Ann. ICRP 31(4).

ICRP, 2003. Biological effects after prenatal irradiation (embryo and fetus). ICRP Publication 90. Ann. ICRP 33(1/2).

ICRP, 2004. Release of patients after therapy with unsealed radionuclides. ICRP Publication 94. Ann. ICRP 34(2).

ICRP, 2007a. The 2007 Recommendations of the International Commission on Radiological Protection. ICRP Publication 103. Ann. ICRP 37(2–4).

ICRP, 2007b. Radiological protection in medicine. ICRP Publication 105. Ann. ICRP 37(6).

ICRP, 2008. Radiation dose to patients from radiopharmaceuticals – Addendum 3 to ICRP Publication 53. ICRP Publication 106. Ann. ICRP 38(1/2).

ICRP, 2009. Education and training in radiological protection for diagnostic and interventional procedures. ICRP Publication 113. Ann. ICRP 39(5).

ICRP, 2010. Conversion coefficients for radiological protection quantities for external radiation exposures. ICRP Publication 116. Ann. ICRP 40(2–5).

ICRP, 2015a. Radiation dose to patients from radiopharmaceuticals: a compendium of current information related to frequently used substances. ICRP Publication 128. Ann. ICRP 44(2S).

ICRP, 2015b. Occupational intakes of radionuclides: Part 1. ICRP Publication 130. Ann. ICRP 44(2).

ICRU, 1993. Quantities and Units in Radiation Protection Dosimetry. ICRU Report 51. International Commission on Radiation Units and Measurements, Bethesda, MD.

ICRU, 2016. Key data for ionizing-radiation dosimetry: measurement standards and applications. ICRU Report No. 90. J. ICRU 14(1).

ISO, 2016. Radiological Protection — Monitoring and Internal Dosimetry for Staff Members Exposed to Medical Radionuclides as Unsealed Sources. ISO 16637. International Organization for Standardization, Geneva.

Ilan, E., Sandstrom, M., Wassberg, C., et al., 2015. Dose response of pancreatic neuroendocrine tumors treated with peptide receptor radionuclide therapy using ^{177}Lu-DOTATATE. J. Nucl. Med. 56, 177–182.

Imhof, A., Brunner, P., Marincek, N., et al., 2011. Response, survival, and long-term toxicity after therapy with the radiolabeled somatostatin analogue [^{90}Y-DOTA]-TOC in metastasized neuroendocrine cancers. J. Clin. Oncol. 29, 2416–2423.

Infante-Rivard, C., Rivard, G.E., Derome, F., et al., 2012. A retrospective cohort study of cancer incidence among patients treated with radiosynoviorthesis. Haemophilia 18, 805–809.

Jarzab, B., Handkiewicz-Junak, D., Wloch, J., 2005. Juvenile differentiated thyroid carcinoma and the role of radioiodine in its treatment: a qualitative review. Endocr-Relat. Cancer 12, 773–803.

Jie, Y., Congjin, L., Xingdang, L., et al., 2013. Efficacy and safety of ^{177}Lu-EDTMP in bone metastatic pain palliation in breast cancer and hormone refractory prostate cancer: a phase II study. Clin. Nucl. Med. 38, 88–92.

Joiner, M.C., van der Kogel, A., 2009. Basic Clinical Radiobiology. CRC Press, Boca Raton, FL.

Johnson, L.S., Yanch, J.C., Shortkroff, S., et al., 1995. Beta-particle dosimetry in radiation synovectomy. Eur. J. Nucl. Med. 22, 977–988.

Jönsson, H., Mattsson, S., 2004. Excess radiation absorbed doses from non-optimised radioiodine treatment of hyperthyroidism. Radiat. Prot. Dosim. 108, 107–111.

Jönsson, L., Ljungberg, M., Strand, S.E., 2005. Evaluation of accuracy in activity calculations for the conjugate view method from Monte Carlo simulated scintillation camera images using experimental data in an anthropomorphic phantom. J. Nucl. Med. 46, 1679–1686.

Jurcic, J.G., Rosenblat, T.L., 2014. Targeted alpha-particle immunotherapy for acute myeloid leukemia. Am. Soc. Clin. Oncol. Educ. Book 34, e126–e131.

Kellerer, A.M., Rossi, H.H., 1974. The theory of dual radiation action. In: Ebert, M., Howard, A. (Eds.), Current Topics in Radiation Research. Vol. III. North Holland Publishing Co., Amsterdam, pp. 85–158.

Klett, R., Puille, M., Matter, H.P., et al., 1999. Activity leakage and radiation exposure in radiation synovectomy of the knee: influence of different therapeutic modalities. Z. Rheumatol. 58, 207–212.

Kletting, P., Schimmel, S., Kestler, H.A., et al., 2013. Molecular radiotherapy: the NUKFIT software for calculating the time-integrated activity coefficient. Med. Phys. 40, 102504.

Klubo-Gwiezdzinska, J., Van Nostrand, D., Burman, K.D., et al., 2010. Salivary gland malignancy and radioiodine therapy for thyroid cancer. Thyroid 20, 647–651.

Knut, L., 2015. Radiosynovectomy in the therapeutic management of arthritis. World J. Nucl. Med. 14, 10–15.

Kobe, C., Eschner, W., Sudbrock, F., et al., 2008. Graves' disease and radioiodine therapy. Is success of ablation dependent on the achieved dose above 200 Gy? Nuklearmedizin 47, 13–17.

Kraeber-Bodere, F., Rousseau, C., Bodet-Milin, C., et al., 2006. Targeting, toxicity, and efficacy of 2-step, pretargeted radioimmunotherapy using a chimeric bispecific antibody and ^{131}I-labeled bivalent hapten in a phase I optimization clinical trial. J. Nucl. Med. 47, 247–255.

Kramer, K., Humm, J.L., Souweidane, M.M., et al., 2007. Phase I study of targeted radioimmunotherapy for leptomeningeal cancer using intra-Ommaya [131]I-3FB. J. Clin. Oncol. 25, 5465–5470.

Kratochwil, C., Bruchertseifer, F., Giesel, F.L., et al., 2016. [225]Ac-PSMA-617 for PSMA-targeted alpha-radiation therapy of metastatic castration-resistant prostate cancer. J. Nucl. Med. 5, 1941–1944.

Kunikowska, J., Krolicki, L., Hubalewska-Dydejczyk, A., et al., 2011. Clinical results of radionuclide therapy of neuroendocrine tumours with ^{90}Y-DOTATATE and tandem ^{90}Y/^{177}Lu-DOTATATE: which is a better therapy option? Eur. J. Nucl. Med. Mol. Imaging 38, 1788–1797.

Kwekkeboom, D.J., Mueller-Brand, J., Paganelli, G., et al., 2005. Overview of results of peptide receptor radionuclide therapy with 3 radiolabeled somatostatin analogs. J. Nucl. Med. 46 (Suppl. 1), 62S–66S.

Lambert, B., Mertens, J., Sturm, E.J., et al., 2010. ^{99m}Tc-labelled macroaggregated albumin (MAA) scintigraphy for planning treatment with ^{90}Y microspheres. Eur. J. Nucl. Med. Mol. Imaging 37, 2328–2333.

Lancelot, S., Guillet, B., Sigrist, S., et al., 2008. Exposure of medical personnel to radiation during radionuclide therapy practices. Nucl. Med. Commun. 29, 405–410.

Larson, S.M., Carrasquillo, J.A., Cheung, N-K., et al., 2015. Radioimmunotherapy of human tumours. Nat. Rev. Cancer 15, 347–360.

Lassmann, M., Hanscheid, H., Chiesa, C., et al., 2008. EANM Dosimetry Committee series on standard operational procedures for pre-therapeutic dosimetry I: blood and bone marrow dosimetry in differentiated thyroid cancer therapy. Eur. J. Nucl. Med. Mol. Imaging 35, 1405–1412.

Lea, D.E., Catcheside, D.G., 1942. The mechanism of the induction by radiation of chromosome aberrations in tradescantia. J. Genet. 44, 216–245.

Lee, S.L., 2010. Complications of radioactive iodine treatment of thyroid carcinoma. J. Natl. Compr. Canc. Netw. 8, 1277–1286; quiz 1287.

Leiter, L., Seidlin, S.M., Marinelli, L.D., 1946. Adenocarcinoma of the thyroid with hyperthyroidism and functional metastases; studies with thiouracil and radioiodine. J. Clin. Endocrinol. Metab. 6, 247–261.

Leslie, W.D., Ward, L., Salamon, E.A., et al., 2003. A randomized comparison of radioiodine doses in Graves' hyperthyroidism. J. Clin. Endocrinol. Metab. 88, 978–983.

Lhommel, R., van Elmbt, L., Goffette, P., et al., 2010. Feasibility of ^{90}Y TOF PET-based dosimetry in liver metastasis therapy using SIR-spheres. Eur. J. Nucl. Med. Mol. Imaging 37, 1654–1962.

Liepe, K., Andreeff, M., Wunderlich, G., et al., 2005a. Radiation protection in radiosynovectomy of the knee. Health Phys. 89, 151–154.

Liepe, K., Runge, R., Kotzerk, J., 2005b. The benefit of bone-seeking radiopharmaceuticals in the treatment of metastatic bone pain. J. Cancer Res. Clin. Oncol. 131, 60–66.

Liepe, K., Kotzerke, J., 2007. A comparative study of [188]Re-HEDP, [186]Re-HEDP, [153]Sm-EDTMP and ^{89}Sr in the treatment of painful skeletal metastases. Nucl. Med. Commun. 28, 623–630.

Ljungberg, M., Celler, A., Konijnenberg, M.W., et al., 2016. MIRD Pamphlet No. 26: joint EANM/MIRD guidelines for quantitative ^{177}Lu SPECT applied for dosimetry of radiopharmaceutical therapy. J. Nucl. Med. 57, 151–162.

Loevinger, R., Berman, M., 1968. A schema for absorbed-dose calculations for biologically distributed radionuclides. MIRD Pamphlet No. 1. J. Nucl. Med. 9 (Suppl. 1), 7–14.

Luster, M., Clarke, S.E., Dietlein, M., et al., 2008. Guidelines for radioiodine therapy of differentiated thyroid cancer. Eur. J. Nucl. Med. Mol. Imaging 35, 1941–1959.

Mallick, U., Harmer, C., Hackshaw, A., et al., 2012a. Iodine or not (IoN) for low-risk differentiated thyroid cancer: the next UK National Cancer Research Network randomised trial following HiLo. Clin. Oncol. 24, 159–161.

Mallick, U., Harmer, C., Yap, B., et al., 2012b. Ablation with low-dose radioiodine and thyrotropin alfa in thyroid cancer. N. Engl. J. Med. 366, 1674–1685.

Matthay, K.K., Panina, C., Huberty, J., et al., 2001. Correlation of tumor and whole-body dosimetry with tumor response and toxicity in refractory neuroblastoma treated with ^{131}I-MIBG. J. Nucl. Med. 42, 1713–1721.

Matthay, K.K., Yanik, G., Messina, J., et al., 2007. Phase II study on the effect of disease sites, age, and prior therapy on response to iodine-131-metaiodobenzylguanidine therapy in refractory neuroblastoma. J. Clin. Oncol. 25, 1054–1060.

Maxon, H.R. 3rd, Englaro, E.E., Thomas, S.R., et al., 1992. Radioiodine-131 therapy for well-differentiated thyroid cancer – a quantitative radiation dosimetric approach: outcome and validation in 85 patients. J. Nucl. Med. 33, 1132–1136.

McKay, E., 2003. A software tool for specifying voxel models for dosimetry estimation. Cancer Biother. Radiopharm. 18, 61–69.

Menda, Y., O'Dorisio, M.S., Kao, S., et al., 2010. Phase I trial of ^{90}Y-DOTATOC therapy in children and young adults with refractory solid tumors that express somatostatin receptors. J. Nucl. Med. 51, 1524–1531.

Merrill, S., Horowitz, J., Traino, A.C., et al., 2011. Accuracy and optimal timing of activity measurements in estimating the absorbed dose of radioiodine in the treatment of Graves' disease. Phys. Med. Biol. 56, 557–571.

Miederer, M., McDevitt, M.R., Sgouros, G., et al., 2004. Pharmacokinetics, dosimetry, and toxicity of the targetable atomic generator, [225]Ac-HuM195, in nonhuman primates. J. Nucl. Med. 45, 129–137.

Millar, W.T., 1991. Application of the linear-quadratic model with incomplete repair to radionuclide directed therapy. Br. J. Radiol. 64, 242–251.

NCRP, 2006. Management of Radionuclide Therapy Patients. NCRP Report No. 155. National Council on Radiation Protection and Measurements, Bethesda, MD.

Noble, J., Jones, A.G., Davies, M.A., et al., 1983. Leakage of radioactive particle systems from a synovial joint studied with a gamma camera: its application to radiation synovectomy. J. Bone Joint Surg. Am. 65, 381–389.

Norrgren, K., Svegborn, S.L., Areberg, J., Mattsson, S., 2003. Accuracy of the quantification of organ activity from planar gamma camera images. Cancer Biother. Radiopharm. 18, 125–131.

Pandit-Taskar, N., Batraki, M., Divgi, C.R., 2004. Radiopharmaceutical therapy for palliation of bone pain from osseous metastases. J. Nucl. Med. 45, 1358–1365.

Pandit-Taskar, N., Larson, S.M., Carrasquillo, J.A., 2014. Bone-seeking radiopharmaceuticals for treatment of osseous metastases. Part 1: alpha therapy with [223]Ra-dichloride. J. Nucl. Med. 55, 268–274.

Parker, C., Nilsson, S., Heinrich, D., et al., 2013. Alpha emitter radium-223 and survival in metastatic prostate cancer. N. Engl. J. Med. 369, 213–223.

Pauwels, S., Barone, R., Walrand, S., et al., 2005. Practical dosimetry of peptide receptor radionuclide therapy with Y-90-labeled somatostatin analogs. J. Nucl. Med. 46, 92S–98S.

Pawelczak, M., David, R., Franklin, B., et al., 2010. Outcomes of children and adolescents with well-differentiated thyroid carcinoma and pulmonary metastases following I-131 treatment: a systematic review. Thyroid 20, 1095–1101.

Perros, P., Boelaert, K., Colley, S., et al., 2014. Guidelines for the management of thyroid cancer. Clin. Endocrinol. 81 (Suppl. 1), 1–122.

Quach, A., Ji, L., Mishra, V., et al., 2011. Thyroid and hepatic function after high-dose ^{131}I-metaiodobenzylguanidine (^{131}I-MIBG) therapy for neuroblastoma. Pediatr. Blood Cancer 56, 191–201.

Rahbar, K., Ahmadzadehfar, H., Kratochwil, C., et al., 2017. German multicenter study investigating ^{177}Lu-PSMA-617 radioligand therapy in advanced prostate cancer patients. J. Nucl. Med. 58, 85–90.

Ramage, J.K., Ahmed, A., Ardill, J., et al., 2012. Guidelines for the management of gastroenteropancreatic neuroendocrine (including carcinoid) tumours (NETs). Gut 61, 6–32.

RCP, 2007. Radioiodine in the Management of Benign Thyroid Disease: Clinical Guidelines. RCP Report of a Working Party. Royal College of Physicians, London.

Reinhardt, M.J., Brink, I., Joe, A.Y., et al., 2002. Radioiodine therapy in Graves' disease based on tissue-absorbed dose calculations: effect of pre-treatment thyroid volume on clinical outcome. Eur. J. Nucl. Med. Mol. Imaging 29, 1118–1124.

Remy, H.L., Borget, I, Leboulleux, S., et al., 2008. [131]I effective half-life and dosimetry in thyroid cancer patients. J. Nucl. Med. 49, 1445–1450.

Rimpler, A., Barth, I., 2007. Beta radiation exposure of medical staff and implications for extremity dose monitoring. Radiat. Prot. Dosim. 125, 335–339.

Rimpler, A., Barth, I., Ferrari, O., et al., 2011. Extremity exposure in nuclear medicine therapy with ^{90}Y-labelled substances – results of the ORAMED project. Radiat. Meas. 46, 1283–1286.

Roedler, H.D., 1980. Accuracy of internal dose calculations with special consideration of radiopharmaceutical biokinetics. In: Watson, E.E., Schlafke-Stelson, A.T., Coffey, J.L., et al. (Eds.), Third International Radiopharmaceutical Symposium. U.S. Department of Human Services, Oak Ridge, TN, pp. 1–20.

Rubino, C., de Vathaire, F., Dottorini, M.E., et al., 2003. Second primary malignancies in thyroid cancer patients. Br. J. Cancer 89, 1638–1644.

Rushforth, D.P., Pratt, B.E., Chittenden, S.J., et al., 2017. InfuShield: a shielded enclosure for administering therapeutic radioisotope treatments using standard syringe pumps. Nucl. Med. Commun. 38, 266–252.

Sans-Merce, M., Ruiz, N., Barth, I., et al., 2011. Recommendations to reduce hand exposure for standard nuclear medicine procedures. Radiat. Meas. 46, 1330–1333.

Savolainen, S., Konijnenberg, M., Bardies, M., et al., 2012. Radiation dosimetry is a necessary ingredient for a perfectly mixed molecular radiotherapy cocktail. Eur. J. Nucl. Med. Mol. Imaging 39, 548–549.

Sawka, A.M., Lea, J., Alshehri, B., et al., 2008a. A systematic review of the gonadal effects of therapeutic radioactive iodine in male thyroid cancer survivors. Clin. Endocrinol. (Oxf.) 68, 610–617.

Sawka, A.M., Lakra, D.C., Lea, J., et al., 2008b. A systematic review examining the effects of therapeutic radioactive iodine on ovarian function and future pregnancy in female thyroid cancer survivors. Clin. Endocrinol. (Oxf.) 69, 479–490.

Schiavo, M., Bagnara, M.C., Calamia, I., et al., 2011. A study of the efficacy of radioiodine therapy with individualized dosimetry in Graves' disease: need to retarget the radiation committed dose to the thyroid. J. Endocrinol. Invest. 34, 201–205.

Schlumberger, M., Catargi, B., Borget, I., et al., 2012. Strategies of radioiodine ablation in patients with low-risk thyroid cancer. N. Engl. J. Med. 366, 1663–1673.

Schmidt, M., Baum, R.P., Simon, T., et al., 2010. Therapeutic nuclear medicine in pediatric malignancy. Q. J. Nucl. Med. Mol. Imaging 54, 411–428.

Seidlin, S.M., Marinelli, L.D., Oshry, E., 1946. Radioactive iodine therapy; effect on functioning metastases of adenocarcinoma of the thyroid. JAMA 132, 838–847.

Seregni, E., Maccauro, M., Chiesa, C., et al., 2014. Treatment with tandem [90Y]DOTA-TATE and [177Lu]DOTA-TATE of neuroendocrine tumours refractory to conventional therapy. Eur. J. Nucl. Med. Mol. Imaging 41, 223–230.

Sgouros, G., Roeske, J.C., McDevitt, M.R., et al., 2010. MIRD Pamphlet No. 22 (abridged): radiobiology and dosimetry of alpha-particle emitters for targeted radionuclide therapy. J. Nucl. Med. 51, 311–328.

Shinto, A.S., Shibu, D., Kamaleshwaran, K.K., et al., 2014. 177Lu-EDTMP for treatment of bone pain in patients with disseminated skeletal metastases. J. Nucl. Med. Technol. 42, 55–61.

Siegel, J.A., Thomas, R., Stubbs, J.R., et al., 1999. MIRD Pamphlet No. 16: techniques for quantitative radiopharmaceutical biodistribution data acquisition and analysis for use in human radiation dose estimates. J. Nucl. Med. 40, 37S–61S.

Silberstein, E.B., Alavi, A., Balon, H.R., et al., 2012. The SNM practice guideline for therapy of thyroid disease with 131I 3.0. J. Nucl. Med. 53, 1633–1651.

Sisson, J.C., Avram, A.M., Rubello, D., et al., 2007. Radioiodine treatment of hyperthyroidism: fixed or calculated doses; intelligent design or science? Eur. J. Nucl. Med. Mol. Imaging 34, 1129–1130.

Sisson, J.C., Freitas, J., McDougall, I.R., et al., 2011. Radiation safety in the treatment of patients with thyroid diseases by radioiodine 131I: practice recommendations of the American Thyroid Association. The American Thyroid Association Taskforce on Radioiodine Safety. Thyroid 21, 335–346.

Smits, M.L., Nijsen, J.F., van den Bosch, M.A., et al., 2012. Holmium-166 radioembolisation in patients with unresectable, chemorefractory liver metastases (HEPAR trial): a phase 1, dose-escalation study. Lancet Oncol. 13, 1025–1034.

Snyder, W.S., Ford, M.R., Warner, G.G., et al., 1969. Estimates of absorbed fractions for monoenergetic photon sources uniformly distributed in various organs of a heterogeneous phantom. MIRD Pamphlet No. 5. J. Nucl. Med. 10 (Suppl. 3), 7–52.

Stabin, M.G., Sparks, R.B., Crowe, E., 2005. OLINDA/EXM: the second-generation personal computer software for internal dose assessment in nuclear medicine. J. Nucl. Med. 46, 1023–1027.

Stokkel, M.P., Handkiewicz, J.D., Lassmann, M., et al., 2010. EANM procedure guidelines for therapy of benign thyroid disease. Eur. J. Nucl. Med. Mol. Imaging 37, 2218–2228.

Strigari, L., Sciuto, R., Rea, S., et al., 2010. Efficacy and toxicity related to treatment of hepatocellular carcinoma with Y-90-SIR spheres: radiobiologic considerations. J. Nucl. Med. 51, 1377–1385.

Strigari, L., Konijnenberg, M., Chiesa, C., et al., 2014. The evidence base for the use of internal dosimetry in the clinical practice of molecular radiotherapy. Eur. J. Nucl. Med. Mol. Imaging 41, 1976–1988.

Strosberg, J., El-Haddad, G., Wolin, E., et al., 2017. Phase 3 trial of ^{177}Lu-dotatate for midgut neuroendocrine tumors. N. Engl. J. Med. 376, 125–135.

Sudbrock, F., Schmidt, M., Simon, T., et al., 2010. Dosimetry for ^{131}I-MIBG therapies in metastatic neuroblastoma, phaeochromocytoma and paraganglioma. Eur. J. Nucl. Med. Mol. Imaging 37, 1279–1290.

Sundlöv, A., Sjögreen-Gleisner, K., Svensson, J., et al., 2017. Individualised ^{177}Lu-DOTATATE treatment of neuroendocrine tumours based on kidney dosimetry. Eur. J. Nucl. Med. Mol. Imaging 44, 1480–1489.

Tennvall, J., Fischer, M., Bischof Delaloye, A., et al., 2007. EANM procedure guideline of radio-immunotherapy for B-cell lymphoma with ^{90}Y-radiolabeled ibritumomab tiuxetan (Zevalin®). Eur. J. Nucl. Med. Mol. Imaging 34, 616–622.

Tennvall, J., Brans, B., 2007. EANM procedure guideline for ^{32}P phosphate treatment of myeloproliferative diseases. Eur. J. Nucl. Med. Mol. Imaging 34, 1324–1327.

Thapa, P., Nikam, D., Das, T., et al., 2015. Clinical efficacy and safety comparison of ^{177}Lu-EDTMP with [153]Sm-EDTMP on an equidose basis in patients with painful skeletal metastases. J. Nucl. Med. 56, 1513–1519.

Tristam, M., Alaamer, A.S., Fleming, J.S., et al., 1996. Iodine-131-metaiodobenzylguanidine dosimetry in cancer therapy: risk versus benefit. J. Nucl. Med. 37, 1058–1063.

Turkmen, C., Ozturk, S., Unal, S.N., et al., 2007. The genotoxic effects in lymphocyte cultures of children treated with radiosynovectomy by using yttrium-90 citrate colloid. Cancer Biother. Radiopharm. 22, 393–399.

Valkema, R., De Jong, M., Bakker, W.H., et al., 2002. Phase I study of peptide receptor radionuclide therapy with [In-DTPA]octreotide: the Rotterdam experience. Semin. Nucl. Med. 32, 110–122.

van der Pol, J., Vöö, S., Bucerius, J., et al., 2017. Consequences of radiopharmaceutical extravasation and therapeutic interventions: a systematic review. Eur. J. Nucl. Med. Mol. Imaging 44, 1234–1243.

Vanhavere, F., Carinon, E., Gualdrini, G., et al., 2012. ORAMED: Optimisation of Radiation Protection for Medical Staff. EURADOS Report 2012-02. European Radiation Dosimetry e. V., Braunschweig.

Vassilopoulou-Sellin, R., Klein, M.J., Smith, T.H., et al., 1993. Pulmonary metastases in children and young adults with differentiated thyroid cancer. Cancer 71, 1348–1352.

Verburg, F.A., Biko, J., Diessl, S., et al., 2011. I-131 activities as high as safely administrable (AHASA) for the treatment of children and adolescents with advanced differentiated thyroid cancer. J. Clin. Endocrinol. Metab. 96, E1268–E1271.

Wagner, H.N. Jr, 2006. A Personal History of Nuclear Medicine. Springer, New York.

Wallace, A.B., Bush, V., 1991. Management and autopsy of a radioactive cadaver. Australas. Phys. Eng. Sci. Med. 14, 119–124.

Walrand, S., Barone, R., Pauwels, S., et al., 2011. Experimental facts supporting a red marrow uptake due to radiometal transchelation in ^{90}Y-DOTATOC therapy and relationship to the decrease of platelet counts. Eur. J. Nucl. Med. Mol. Imaging 38, 1270–1280.

Watson, E.E., Stabin, M.G., Eckerman, K.F., 1989. A model of the peritoneal cavity for use in internal dosimetry. J. Nucl. Med. 30, 2002–2011.

Weiss, B., Vora, A., Huberty, J., et al., 2003. Secondary myelodysplastic syndrome and leukemia following ^{131}I-metaiodobenzylguanidine therapy for relapsed neuroblastoma. J. Pediatr. Hematol. Oncol. 25, 543–547.

Wessels, B.W., Konijnenberg, M.W., Dale, R.G., et al., 2008. MIRD Pamphlet No. 20: the effect of model assumptions on kidney dosimetry and response – implications for radionuclide therapy. J. Nucl. Med. 49, 1884–1899.

Willowson, K.P., Tapner, M., Team, Q.I., et al., 2015. A multicentre comparison of quantitative ^{90}Y PET/CT for dosimetric purposes after radioembolization with resin microspheres: the QUEST phantom study. Eur. J. Nucl. Med. Mol. Imaging 42, 1202–1222.

Wiseman, G.A., White, C.A., Sparks, R.B., et al., 2001. Biodistribution and dosimetry results from a phase III prospectively randomized controlled trial of Zevalin radioimmunotherapy for low-grade, follicular, or transformed B-cell non-Hodgkin's lymphoma. Crit. Rev. Oncol. Hematol. 39, 181–194.

Yousefnia, H., Zolghadri, S., Jalilian, A.R., 2015. Absorbed dose assessment of ^{177}Lu-zoledronate and ^{177}Lu-EDTMP for humans based on biodistribution data in rats. J. Med. Phys. 40, 102–108.

Zanzonico, P.B., Siegel, J.A., St. Germain, J., 2000. A generalized algorithm for determining the time of release and the duration of post-release radiation precautions following radionuclide therapy. Health Phys. 78, 648–659.

Zimmerman, B.E., Grosev, D., Buvat, I., et al., 2017. Multi-centre evaluation of accuracy and reproducibility of planar and SPECT image quantification: an IAEA phantom study. Z. Med. Phys. 27, 98–112.

GLOSSARY

Absorbed dose, D

The quotient of the mean energy (d) imparted to an element of matter by ionising radiation and the mass (dm) of the element.

$$D = \frac{\mathrm{d}\bar{\varepsilon}}{\mathrm{d}m}$$

Absorbed dose is the basic physical dose quantity and is applicable to all types of ionising radiation and to any material. The unit of absorbed dose is $\mathrm{J\,kg}^{-1}$, and its special name is gray (Gy).

Ambient dose equivalent, $H^*(10)$

The dose equivalent at a point in a radiation field that would be produced by the corresponding expanded and aligned field in the ICRU sphere at a depth of 10 mm on the radius opposing the direction of the aligned field. The unit of ambient dose equivalent is $\mathrm{J\,kg}^{-1}$, and its special name is sievert (Sv).

Biologically effective dose (BED)

A concept within the linear-quadratic cell survival model used to calculate the different absorbed doses required to produce the same probability of a specified biological endpoint, when the absorbed doses are delivered with different fractionation schemes or absorbed dose rate patterns. Theoretically, BED is the absorbed dose that would be required to produce a specified biological endpoint if the dose was delivered by infinitesimally small dose fractions or at a very low dose rate.

Comforters and carers

Individuals, other than staff, who care for and comfort patients. These individuals include parents and others, normally family members or close friends, who hold children during diagnostic procedures or may be close to patients following the administration of radiopharmaceuticals or during brachytherapy (ICRP, 2007a).

Deterministic effect

Injury in populations of cells, characterised by a threshold dose and an increase in the severity of the reaction as the dose is increased further. Deterministic effect is also termed a 'tissue reaction'. In some cases, deterministic effects are modifiable by postirradiation procedures including biological response modifiers (ICRP, 2007a).

Dose constraint

A prospective and source-related restriction on the individual dose from a source, which provides a basic level of protection for the most highly exposed individuals from a source, and serves as an upper bound on the dose in optimisation of protection for that source. For occupational exposures, the dose constraint is a value of individual dose used to limit the range of options considered in the process of optimisation. For public exposure, the dose constraint is an upper bound on the annual doses that members of the public should receive from the planned operation of any controlled source.

Dose equivalent, H

The product of D and Q at a point in tissue, where D is the absorbed dose and Q is the quality factor for the specific radiation at this point, thus:

$$H = D \cdot Q$$

The unit of dose equivalent is $J\,kg^{-1}$, and its special name is sievert (Sv).

Dose limit

The value of the effective dose received by an individual within a specified period from planned exposure situations that shall not be exceeded. Dose limitation is one of three fundamental principles of radiological protection originally defined by ICRP.

Effective dose, E

The tissue-weighted sum of the equivalent doses in all specified tissues and organs of the body, given by the expression:

$$E = \sum_T w_T \sum_R w_R D_{T,R}$$

where $D_{T,R}$ is the mean absorbed dose from radiation R in a tissue or organ, T, w_T is the tissue weighting factor, and w_R is the radiation weighting factor.

The unit for effective dose is the same as for absorbed dose ($J\,kg^{-1}$), and its special name is sievert (Sv).

Effective half-life

The time required for the activity of radionuclide deposited in a living organism to be reduced by half as a result of combined action of radioactive decay and biological elimination. The effective half-life, T_{eff}, can be calculated from the corresponding biological half-life, T_i, and the physical half-life, T_p:

$$\frac{1}{T_{eff}} = \frac{1}{T_i} + \frac{1}{T_p}$$

Equivalent dose, H_T

The dose in a tissue or organ T given by:

$$H_T = \sum_R W_R D_{T,R}$$

where $D_{T,R}$ is the mean absorbed dose from radiation R in a tissue or organ T, and w_R is the radiation weighting factor. Since w_R is dimensionless, the unit for the equivalent dose is the same as for absorbed dose, $J\,kg^{-1}$.

Justification

One of three fundamental principles of radiological protection originally defined by ICRP. The process of determining whether: (1) a planned activity involving radiation is beneficial overall (whether the benefits to individuals and to society from introducing or continuing the activity outweigh the harm resulting from the activity); or (2) the decision to control exposure in an emergency or existing exposure situation is likely to be beneficial overall (i.e. whether the benefits to individuals and society outweigh its cost and any harm or damage it causes).

Linear energy transfer (LET)

The average linear energy loss of charged particle radiation in a medium (i.e. the radiation energy lost per unit length of path through a material). That is, the quotient of dE by dl where dE is the mean energy lost by a charged particle owing to collisions with electrons in traversing a distance dl in matter.

$$L = \frac{dE}{dl}$$

The unit of L is $J\,m^{-1}$, often given in $keV\,\mu m^{-1}$.

Occupational exposure

All exposure incurred by workers in the course of their work, with the exception of: (1) excluded exposures and exposures from exempt activities involving radiation or exempt sources; (2) any medical exposure; and (3) the normal local natural background radiation.

Optimisation of protection

The principle of optimisation of radiological protection is a source-related process that aims to keep the magnitude of individual doses, the number of people exposed, and the likelihood of potential exposure as low as reasonably achievable below the appropriate dose criteria (constraint or reference level), economic and societal factors being taken into account.

Organ at risk

Organs that might be damaged during exposure to radiation. This term most frequently refers to healthy organs located in the radiation field during radiotherapy.

Quality factor, $Q(L)$

The factor characterising the biological effectiveness of a radiation, based on the ionisation density along the tracks of ion beams in tissue. Q is defined as a function of the unrestricted linear energy transfer, L_∞ (often denoted as L or LET), of ion beams in water:

$$
Q(L) = \begin{cases} 1 & L < 10\,\text{keV}/\mu\text{m} \\ 0.32L - 2.2 & 10 \leq L \leq 100\,\text{keV}/\mu\text{m} \\ 300/\sqrt{L} & L > 100\,\text{keV}/\mu\text{m} \end{cases}
$$

Q has been replaced by the radiation weighting factor used in calculating effective dose, but is still used in calculating the operational dose equivalent quantities used in monitoring.

Radiation detriment

A concept used to quantify the harmful health effects of radiation exposure in different parts of the body. It is defined by ICRP as a function of several factors, including incidence of radiation-related cancer or heritable effects, lethality of these conditions, quality of life, and years of life lost due to these conditions.

Radiation weighting factor, w_R

A dimensionless factor by which the organ or tissue absorbed dose is weighted to reflect the higher biological effectiveness of high-LET radiations compared with low-LET radiations.

Relative biological effectiveness (RBE)

The ratio of absorbed dose of a low-LET reference radiation to absorbed dose of the radiation considered that gives an identical biological effect. RBE values vary with absorbed dose, dose rate, and biological endpoint considered.

Risk

Risk relates to the probability that a detriment outcome may occur. Relative risk is the rate of disease in an exposed population divided by the rate of disease in an unexposed population. Excess relative risk is the rate of disease in an exposed population divided by the rate of disease in an unexposed population minus 1.0, often expressed as the excess relative risk per sievert (Sv).

Stochastic effect

The induction of malignant disease or heritable effects for which the probability of an effect occurring, but not its severity, is regarded for the purpose of radiological protection to be increasing with the dose without a threshold.

Tissue weighting factor, w_T

The factor by which the equivalent dose to a tissue or organ T is weighted to represent the relative contribution of that tissue or organ to the total health detriment resulting from uniform irradiation of the body (ICRP, 2007b). The factor is weighted such that:

$$\sum_T w_T = 1$$

Voxel phantom

A computational anthropomorphic phantom based on medical tomographic images for which the anatomy is described by small, three-dimensional volume elements (voxels) specifying the density and the atomic composition of the various organs and tissues of the human body.

ACKNOWLEDGEMENTS

Although ICRP has a number of publications on the use of radiopharmaceuticals, this is the first publication specific to radiopharmaceutical therapy. At its meeting in Bethesda, MD, USA in 2011, Committee 3 discussed the need for a publication on this subject, and established a working party to undertake preparatory work. The Main Commission launched Task Group 101 on Radiological Protection in Therapy with Radiopharmaceuticals in 2016.

ICRP thanks all those involved in the development of this publication for their hard work and dedication over many years.

Task Group 101 members *(2016–2019)*

Y. Yonekura (Chair)	C. Divgi[*]	S. Palm[*]
S. Mattsson (Co-Chair)	M. Doruff[*]	P. Zanzonico[*]
W.E. Bolch	D.R. Fisher[*]	
L.T. Dauer	M. Hosono[*]	
G. Flux	M. Lassmann[*]	

[*]Corresponding members.

Committee 3 working party members *(2011–2016)*

Y. Yonekura (Co-chair)	C. Divgi[*]	M. Lassmann[*]
S. Mattsson (Co-Chair)	D.R. Fisher[*]	S. Palm[*]
W.E. Bolch	G. Flux[*]	P. Zanzonico[*]
L.T. Dauer	M. Hosono[*]	

[*]Corresponding members.

Committee 3 critical reviewers

K. Kang	C.J. Martin

Main Commission critical reviewers

C. Cousins	J. Harrison

Editorial members

C.H. Clement (Scientific Secretary and *Annals of the ICRP* Editor-in-Chief)
H. Fujita (Assistant Scientific Secretary and *Annals of the ICRP* Associate Editor)
(2018–)
H. Ogino (Assistant Scientific Secretary and *Annals of the ICRP* Associate Editor)
(2016–2018)

Committee 3 members during preparation of this publication

(2009–2013)

E. Vañó (Chair)	I. Gusev	H. Ringert
J-M. Cosset (Vice-Chair)	J.W. Hopewell	M. Rosenstein
M. Rehani (Secretary)	P-L. Khong	Y. Yonekura
K. Åhlström Riklund	S. Mattsson	B. Yue
M.R. Baeza	D.L. Miller	
L.T. Dauer	P. Ortiz López	

(2013–2017)

E. Vañó (Chair)	L.T. Dauer	P. Ortiz López
D.L. Miller (Vice-Chair)	S. Demeter	P. Scalliet
M. Rehani (Secretary)	K. Kang	Y. Yonekura
K. Åhlström Riklund	P-L. Khong	B. Yue
K. Applegate	R. Loose	
M. Bourguignon	C.J. Martin	

(2017–2021)

K. Applegate (Chair)	M.C. Cantone	J.M. Marti-Climent
C.J. Martin (Vice-Chair)	S. Demeter	Y. Niu
M. Rehani (Secretary)	M. Hosono	W. Small
J.S. Alsuwaidi	K. Kang	D. Sutton
M. Bourguignon	R. Loose	L. Van Bladel

Committee 3 emeritus members

S. Mattsson	M. Rosenstein

Main Commission members at the time of approval of this publication

ICRP and the members of Task Group 101 thank Katarina Sjögreen Gleisner for her valuable contribution to this publication.

Finally, thank you very much to all organisations and individuals who took the time to provide comments on the the draft of this publication during the consultation process.

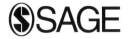
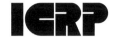

CORRIGENDUM

Corrigendum to ICRP *Publication 128*: Radiation dose to patients from radiopharmaceuticals: a compendium of current information related to frequently used substances. [Ann. ICRP 44(2S), 2015]. DOI: 10.1177/0146645314558019.

The following error has been identified in Table C.109, p. 280:

The value of the absorbed dose per unit activity administered to the urinary bladder wall for the 1-year-old child after oral administration of ^{131}I-iodide should be $1.3E + 00$ mGy MBq^{-1}, not 1.3E-01 as was originally stated.

ICRP apologises for any inconvenience or confusion caused by this error.

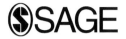

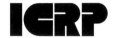

CORRIGENDUM

Corrigendum to ICRP *Publication 128*: Radiation dose to patients from radiopharmaceuticals: a compendium of current information related to frequently used substances. [Ann. ICRP 44(2S), 2015]. DOI: 10.1177/0146645314558019.

The following error has been identified in Table C.109, p. 280 (oral administration of ^{131}I-iodide, patients with high uptake in the thyroid):

The absorbed dose to the testes per unit activity administered should be 2.2E-02 mGy MBq^{-1} for the adult, not 2.2E-01 as was originally stated.

ICRP apologises for any inconvenience or confusion caused by this error.

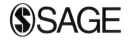
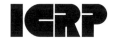

CORRIGENDUM

Corrigendum to ICRP *Publication 139*: Occupational radiological protection in interventional procedures [Ann. ICRP 47(2), 2018]. DOI: 10.1177/0146645317750356.

Some figures in Table 4.1 were incorrect. The corrected figures appear in bold italic in the table below.

ICRP apologises for any inconvenience or confusion caused by these errors.

Table 4.1. α and β values [adapted from Järvinen et al. (2008)] of the algorithms that best meet the criteria of no underestimation and minimum overestimation for the typical geometries, and an algorithm based on *Publication 103* (ICRP, 2007a) weighting factors for effective dose.

	With thyroid shielding		Without thyroid shielding	
Algorithm	α	β	α	β
Swiss Ordinance (2008)	1	0.05	1	0.1
McEwan (2000)			0.71	0.05
Von Boetticher et al. (2010)	*0.84*	0.051	*0.79*	0.100

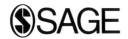
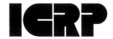

CORRIGENDUM

Corrigendum to ICRP *Publication 139*: Occupational radiological protection in interventional procedures. [Ann. ICRP 47(2), 2018]. DOI: 10.1177/0146645317750356.

An error has been identified in the following equation in Annex B, Paragraph B9, p. 116:

$$E = \sum_{T} w_{\mathrm{T}} H_{\mathrm{T}} = \sum_{T} w_{\mathrm{T}} \sum_{T} w_{\mathrm{T}} D_{\mathrm{T,R}}$$

In this equation, the second summation should be over R rather than T

$$E = \sum_{T} w_{\mathrm{T}} H_{\mathrm{T}} = \sum_{T} w_{\mathrm{T}} \sum_{R} w_{\mathrm{R}} D_{\mathrm{T,R}}$$

ICRP apologises for any inconvenience or confusion caused by this error.

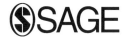 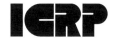

CORRIGENDUM

Corrigendum to Proceedings of the Fourth International Symposium on the System of Radiological Protection [Ann. ICRP 47(3/4), 2018]. DOI: 10.1177/0146645318759619.

On the title page, Associate Editors should be H. OGINO, N. HAMADA, and H. FUJITA.

In addition, the following acknowledgement was erroneously omitted from the Editorial, and should appear immediately before the paragraph beginning 'Most importantly, . . .':

'Preparation of the proceedings of each symposium is also an enormous task. For this, very many thanks to: the authors who submitted papers and reviewed proofs; Haruyuki Ogino and Nobuyuki Hamada who joined me on the Proceedings Editorial Board; the anonymous peer reviewers; Associate Editor Hiroki Fujita who managed the completion of the proceedings issue; and ICRP Interns Julie Reyjal, Laila Omar-Nazir, and Braedon Carr who helped in many ways.'

Annals of the ICRP Editor-in-Chief Christopher H. Clement apologises for any inconvenience or confusion caused by these omissions.

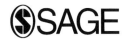 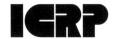

ADDENDUM

Addendum to The International Commission on Radiological Protection at 90 [Ann. ICRP 47(3/4), pp. 343–413]. DOI: 10.1177/0146645318795909.

Too late to include in this paper, new information came to light on a meeting of the International X-ray and Radium Protection Commission held in 1931. Had this been known, Table 1 would have included a row for 1931 indicating that no Chairman was specified for that meeting, and that George W.C. Kaye and Stanley Melville were the Secretaries.

In addition, the following would have been added between the entries for 1928 and 1934 on p. 389:

1931 International X-ray and Radium Protection Commission

At the Third International Congress of Radiology, Paris

Gustav Grossman (Germany)
René Ledoux-Lebard (France)
Rolf M. Sievert (Sweden)
Iser Solomon (France)
Lauriston S. Taylor (USA)
Enzo Pugno-Vanoni (Italy)
George W.C. Kaye, Honorary Secretary (UK)
Stanley Melville, Honorary Secretary (UK)

Source

ICR, 1931. The work of the International X-ray Unit Committee and the International X-ray and Radium Protection Commission during the III International Congress of Radiology in Paris 1931. Acta Radiol. 12, 586–594.